My Parents and Alzheimer's

My Parents and Alzheimer's

A Daughter's Story

Janet M. Stone

VANTAGE PRESS
New York

Published by Vantage Press, Inc.
516 West 34th Street, New York, New York 10001

Manufactured in the United States of America
ISBN: 0-533-13551-6

Library of Congress Catalog Card No.: 00-91320

0 9 8 7 6 5 4 3 2

I want to thank my family for helping me through the difficult years described in this book. I love you all very much.

Acknowledgments

I would like to acknowledge the extraordinary debt I owe to the nurses who cared for my parents.

I could not have written this book without the help of Nancy Mellon, author and teacher, who clearly understood my intention. Her insight inspired me to crucial new perspectives. Nancy is the founding director of a School of Therapeutic Storytelling in the U.S.

I am grateful to Deanna Feenstra who was always eager to read my next page, freshly off the computer.

Thanks to all my friends who valued my belief that giving up outside activity for sake of the completion of my book was a worthwhile choice.

With deep affection I am grateful to my children who did not impose their needs on me while I was writing this book, and for their faithfulness and love toward their grandparents.

Gordon, my husband and guardian angel, often believes in me more than I do myself. If the angels in heaven are as supportive as you are, Gordon, we have nothing to fear.

Preface

For six years I became the primary caretaker of my parents and their home. I cannot recall another time in my life that filled me with such exhaustion and, ironically, such pure energy and joy. My parents were unusual in taking a very positive attitude toward the dying process. I was inspired by them to be totally committed and resourceful during the final years of their lives. I feel moved to tell our story because I want people to know that it is possible to transform tragedy into vibrant life. I want to challenge my readers to see the resources that are stored within them to help face death.

Although I have a fine memory, I kept journals throughout those caregiving years, as I had all my life. I also used a tape recorder in order to get some distance and perspective on my conflicting thoughts and feelings.

When I decided to write this book I sat on the couch one day and imagined what my parents would have thought.

I began with my mother. I imagined visiting her in the living room. She was sitting across from me in her usual chair. "Mother, I want to write a book about our experience with Alzheimer's disease, but I am concerned you might not like everyone knowing our family business."

Her answer was brisk and clear: "What do I care? Everyone I know is already dead."

I turned and envisioned my father seated in his wing-back chair. "Daddy, you had a disease called Alzheimer's. I would like to write a book explaining our family's experience with this disease, but I feel I need your permission because much of it will be about you."

"Do you know what you're talking about?" he asked.

"Yes."

"Are there people out there who really need to hear what you have to say?"

"Definitely," I answered.

"Well then, what are you doing here talking to me? Go write it!"

Writing this book has been a long, vigorous five-year expedition in self-knowledge. I rented an office and went to work every day. I created an island of peace and let go of other things I might have been doing. I wanted to put myself and my experience to the best possible use. My horns locked, and I kept going. I feel grateful and satisfied that this has been possible.

Atkinson, New Hampshire
June 1999

My Parents and Alzheimer's

1

Life is difficult.

—Scott Peck

My mother was dying and my father was showing signs of Alzheimer's disease. It was December 1986 and my life had taken on new responsibilities. Facing illness and death became all-consuming. I cannot recall another time in my life that filled me with such exhaustion and such energy and joy.

I grew up in Haverhill, thirty miles north of Boston, bordering New Hampshire. Full-grown maples gracefully lined the street of my childhood home and the neighborhood of generous single-family dwellings. On Eastland Terrace my sister and I each had our own bedroom. It was considered modern when my parents added a bathroom off theirs. Our driveway was wide, with a circular turn-around at the end. My father always tooted three times before driving in. My mother left the back door open, listening for scraped knees. When the trees were young the houses had awnings to keep out the summer sun. Flower boxes rested beneath each windowsill; hedges of cut-flower beds and bridal-wreath shrubs bordered each neighbor's yard. Hot summer evenings my sister and I would sleep on gliders in the screened porch, waiting patiently to be frightened by lightning bugs. Moving vans were strangers to the area, and the milkman, the iceman, the vegetable man flourished along with the egg man, the garbage man, the grocery man, the fish man, and the ice-cream man. My mother loved her home. My father loved his work. He never tried to run her business, and she never interfered in his. This agreement was their love pact, which endured for sixty-nine years.

In my childhood all our meals were served in the dining room. I sat at the opposite end of the table facing my father, my mother stationed herself in front of the swinging door leading into the kitchen, and my sister Barbara, faced the outside windows. We had dinner every evening except on Sunday, when my mother prepared the 1:30 P.M. ritual Sunday dinner and my father prepared supper, usually a choice of western sandwich, with or without onion, or cold kidney beans with sliced red onion on dark Roman Meal or white Wonder bread. The Sabbath was a family day; there was no going to the movies or playing over at a friend's house. Barbara and I were also limited to the length of time we spent on the phone. Every Sunday night we played Go to the Head of the Class and Pollyanna. Then Mother would help me shampoo my hair in the kitchen sink. When I was early grammar school age I would lean over the sink as she poured glasses full of water to rinse the suds from my hair, adding cider vinegar to the rinse water. Later, when high technology was introduced into the kitchen, she rinsed the soap with chrome nozzle spray gun attached to the sink. When I was older I rinsed my hair with fresh lemon, hoping to make my brown hair blond. While I sat on the living room couch, setting my hair, with pink rollers, bobby pins, and a light blue hair net piled in my lap, we watched the famous "Ed Sullivan Show." I still remember all the hoopla over the Beatles, the already-famous group from Liver-

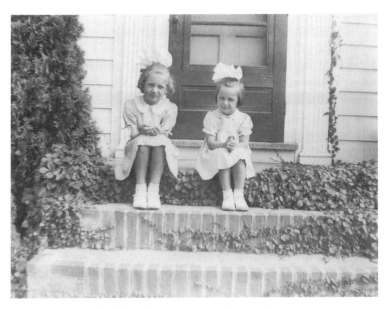
My older sister Barbara with me in 1942

pool, England, who had arrived to entertain us here in America, as though England were light-years away.

By age ten I had learned that being tired was a weakness and being lazy was out of the question. On more than one occasion I heard my father say, "Tired, what's that? I have never been tired a day in my life." In 1956 my parents added a family room to the back of their house. Mother asked my father what style couch he would like to have. "Who needs a couch?" he said, "If someone's so tired they need to lie down then they belong in bed."

My mother was as surefooted regarding her household responsibilities as my father was in valuing his community obligations. Alice was a homemaker, with a wardrobe of house dresses. At four o'clock each day she

3

changed into her afternoon habit, applied lipstick and put on her apron. She was never a club lady, although she supported the Haverhill City Club and the Hale Hospital Auxiliary by carrying a lifetime membership card. She never drove an automobile, although she did have a license, which she used for identification purposes only. She was a very wiry person, and I never remember her asking my father to open a jar. She put out her own ash barrels almost as big as she was and rinsed them weekly, along with the garbage can. Mother was in charge with grit and determination. Nothing got in the way of her spring housecleaning routine. She tired by the end of the day, but she wouldn't want to stop her housework early in order to change her clothes and freshen up. She wouldn't accept my father's dinner invitation to a local restaurant. A shopping trip to Boston was out of the question. She would strip the house to its bare bones, starting upstairs in their bedroom. With the red-handled paintbrush she kept in the bottom drawer she touched up the windowsills with Benjamin Moore white linen, covering up chipped spots where the winter frost had caused the paint to lift. She never would give you any warning as to whether your closet would be washed down or freshly painted. I never liked the idea of her stripping my closet while I was at school. It felt like an invasion of privacy, something I would never do with my own children. Mother saved the turning of mattresses until I got home from school at 3:15 P.M. and we could do it together.

Her three-week cleaning ritual always ended on a Thursday near four o'clock, the day before her standard Friday morning hairdresser appointment, just in time to start dinner. There were many signs her mission was complete. The house smelled unusually fresh. Because the window shades had not been pulled down to the halfway mark, cleanliness stared wide-eyed at you. The bucket containing her cleaning supplies sat orderly at the cellar door. I can see her in the kitchen now ironing the starched doilies she had sprinkled and rolled the day before with no lipstick, her nails, usually polished with Revlon's Windsor, chipped, and her hands red and chapped from ammonia and water solution. A hanky was rolled under the cuff of her light gray cardigan. As a child I thought she looked sour, but now I understand how tired she must have felt. Making a clean home for her family was my mother's gift of love. She always overdid it. By the following week she would often be running to the john for three days and needing smelling salts. Yet, her devotion to the household never faltered. Saturday afternoons at two o'clock my mother would give herself a weekly facial and stretch out on her mahogany twin bed. I am thankful for her example.

In the 1930s it was customary for middle-class families to employ "mother's helpers," Doja came to live with us at eighteen and stayed for ten years. After I married, every few months, I visited Doja; I would bring dinner and we would reminisce. When she was eighty and lived alone in an apartment at a senior complex I asked if she would give me a sketch of what it was like living with my family in those early years. She smiled and said, "It is hard to believe I once was so shy I hid beside your mother's stove when guests dropped in."

Doja was twelve when she started hiring out to help mothers. She was from a large family, had one dress, and was fed up with not having more. She liked my mother the first moment she met her. Doja had been graciously welcomed by my father the Thursday night she went to get hired. "Doja, come on in," he had said. From the start she felt like one of the family, as though she had found a home with my parents. She could laugh, have fun, and be herself. Although she was shy and would have preferred to eat alone, they insisted she be included. She had her own room on the third floor that my parents had made for her; girls who lived in with other families slept in with the daughter. The room was made to look pretty. There were twin maple beds on either side of the window and an attic fan if she needed it. There was a vanity with a chair. My mother was good to her. Never did she go to Boston without bringing her something back. Sometimes it was a dress; one time she brought her back a ring that changed stones. My mother had seen an ad in the Sunday paper, and she knew Doja would like it.

My mother and Doja were a couple of nuts when it came to cleaning. They were both hard workers and committed to the art of housework. Mother always seemed surprised that Doja could work so hard. She never got angry at her when she didn't approve of her actions, even when her big bare feet hung out when she washed windows or when she broke the ball off the top of the fireplace andirons. One spring Doja thought she would help put the storm windows down in the cellar. She stacked the small windows on top of the big ones. When my father came home and saw they had all cracked and broken he just laughed: "Doja, don't try to save us money." My mother had a temper, but she kept it down.

Doja told me that my mother had a very difficult time getting in the family way. I knew my parents were married fifteen years before my elder sister was born. The day my mother went into the hospital to give birth to me she had a cold and they gave her ether. Afterward they wouldn't let her come home. My parents handed me over to Doja. My mother never cried much, but that day she came home from her three-week stay in the hospital Doja

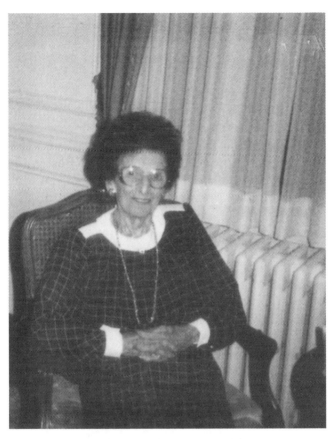
My mother Alice Marble in 1986

found her crying in the living room. Doja put her arm around her and said, "Don't let him see you crying or he'll think, you're not well enough and send you upstairs to rest." Over the next few days my mother's situation got worse. The odor in the house was awful. At first they thought it was me and kept changing me. Every time

Doja brought me in to see my mother she'd say, "Doja, I think the baby needs to be changed." Then Doja began to think, *Is it me or Alice?* the only one they didn't question was my father.

"Your father was not a man who wasted time," Doja joked. By the second day he had called Dr. Armitage and arranged it so they could take X rays in the bedroom. They discovered my mother had an abscess on her lung. She was moved to the Baker Hospital of Boston, where she remained for nearly ten months. I listened intently to Doja as though a window shade were being lifted partway, casting light on my earliest experiences. As an adult I understood that if children do not have the comfort and security of parental care, they need to learn to compensate for this loss. Though I had a nurturing replacement, I can only assume that my mother's absence added to my determination to be with her. I didn't get her when I was a baby, but I was sure-shooting going to be with her at the end.

It was not unusual for me to hear my father described as a devoted man. But hearing it once again from Doja explained how he was like that from the start. My father went into Boston every day to visit my mother and found ways to have dinner with my sister at night. In between he worked and built a business. Once a week Doja went along and brought me in. This way my mother was able to keep up with what was going on. It was Doja's day off, the first she had taken in several months. My father was caring for both me and my sister. Doja left him her telephone number just in case he needed her. She received a call and sensed he was very worried, so she returned to the house. She thought it was the spinach I ate that caused my discomfort that day. Before she left home she told him to give me a quarter-teaspoon of castor oil. A half hour later I was fine. My father couldn't get over it. He got a kick out of things, and this was one of them. Doja remembered him saying, "Imagine how smart that fellow must have been to come up with a remedy where only one-quarter of a teaspoon could do the trick?"

I was still in grammar school the first time I became aware of my mother fainting. It was during the seven o'clock hour, just before my bedtime. I was seated on the couch in my pink robe with matching pink quilted slippers with petite satin ribbons. My mother was seated in her favorite wingback chair, engrossed in her daily ritual of reading the *Haverhill Gazette;* my father was smoking his pipe and thumbing a trade magazine; my sister and I were seated on the couch sorting through and swapping magazine photos of movie stars we had been collecting over the years. Our cousin Sandy would be bringing her assortment of photos to our clean house on Sunday, and we would spend hours spread across my bed swapping memorabilia the same way people exchange baseball cards now. Mother's head tipped forward and the newspaper fell into her lap. At first, I thought she had dozed off until I saw my father jump from his chair, instructing me to get my mother's purse from the drawer in the credenza. I knew just where I was supposed to go because that was where she always kept her pocketbook until she brought it upstairs with her at night just before retiring. With concern in his eyes he turned and said calmly, "Janet, unzip that little pocket along the inside. You will find some smelling salts; hand them to me." I had never seen anything like it before. He slowly passed the salts back and forth like a pendulum underneath my mother's nose. The moment she jerked upward he discarded the gauze capsule in the dish sitting next to her chair. Later I came to understand that Mother's fainting spells had incurred during her period of recovery from her giving her all.

While my mother took care of the household details my father made tireless efforts to satisfy his customers at his automobile dealership. He dressed for his customers, wearing the finest shoes. These silent messages were intended to be reassuring gestures of respect. He wanted people to notice them. The economic structure of Haverhill was made up of many multigenerational businesses. Haverhill's shoe-manufacturing industry had earned it the title of Queen Shoe City of the World. His clientele was buying the top of the market in automobiles; by wearing expensive hand-stitched shoes, he was complimenting them on their ability to identify quality and their good taste in fine cars. My father was a people person. He was directed and had purpose to his conversation.

Gracious and charming, my father also was a bulldozer. He would chew out people who complained about paying taxes by quipping, "What do you care if your taxes are too high? Worry instead about the day you don't have to pay any." At my father's funeral, Charlie Hurwitz said how if my father didn't agree with you he would simply say, "You don't know what you're talking about." For my father, when something was right it was right, period.

My father included in his ethical system a positive attitude toward my mistakes. Like all self-made men, he allowed himself a close bond with trial and error. When I was a child my father did not punish me for my mistakes. Instead he used lecture and reason to correct misconduct. In my case the issue was usually a report card with many unsatisfactory checks in conduct and self-control. The problem in school was never mentioned at the dinner table. He would wait until my bedtime and call me into the kitchen, where we spoke alone. Most often he would use the typical "you're not hurting me; you're hurting yourself" approach. The ending of these lectures was predictable and unique: "Let's have a glass of milk and change the subject before you go to bed." My father was stern, he was a negotiator, he was a fighter, but he had somehow learned the art of knowing when to let go. Later, as his Alzheimer's progressed, I saw this in his expression of relinquishment and resignation.

Our six-year journey began on Monday, December 15, 1986. I usually visited my mother on Mondays. My father would be at work at his auto dealership, where my husband, Gordon, and my brother-in-law John also worked. Mother would be glad to be alone and settling into her weekly routine. She loved routine. My parents lived one mile north from where I lived with my husband and three children. My sister lived one mile south of my parents' house with her husband and four children. Visiting Mother was easy. She was eighty-six and not interested in being either argumentative or judgmental. Our visits carried the aroma of sweet honeysuckle, even now, I think of my mother and our visits during those difficult years every time I smell the honeysuckle bush in our side yard.

As I approached my parents' driveway that morning at nine-thirty, I was surprised to see Lori's car. Lori usually cleaned on Thursday. Mother often referred to her as her "right hand man." *Oh well*, I thought, *Mother will be glad to see her no matter what day it is.* Because my parent's back door opened directly into their kitchen, I immediately noticed Mother sitting quietly in her rocking chair and Lori a few feet away dusting the chrome along the edges of the stove. Why didn't Lori have her boom box blasting out her favorite music? And why was Mother *sitting* at this time of day? I started to say hello, but Lori's eyes pulled me in. "Are you all right, Mother?" I asked. I questioned the yellowish tinge on her face. Was it shadow or was she jaundiced?

"I don't know," she replied. "I was just sitting here trying to figure that out myself."

I looked at Lori and asked, "Do you think I should call the doctor?"

She answered, using a blunt tone, "I think you should call your father and tell him to call the doctor." My father clearly saw mother as his responsibility and would have been incensed if I interfered. My fear kicked in the moment I glanced out Mother's dining room window and saw my father's car round the corner into the driveway.

I wanted to watch my mother closely while we drove to the hospital. That is why I sat in the backseat behind my father, from where I was able to view her profile. I asked myself, *What is causing my shaking? Is it his driving or is it his solicitous repetitive questioning?* My mother's cheeks quivering while her lips moved back and forth, pressing against each other. I felt so helpless. Whenever I tried to relieve some of her tension by answering my father's questions, he'd interrupt with, "Be quiet. I didn't ask you; I asked your mother. I want to hear what she has to say." I wanted to yell, "Be quite and leave her alone," but I had never spoken back to my father. It was then, in the backseat of his luxury sedan, I felt that no one has a right to get away with being unreasonable, regardless of their age or good intentions. This realization became increasing important to me during the next six years.

Three miles away at the Hale Hospital, the doctor guided my father and me around the corner to a quiet section and gestured for us to take a seat. My father refused. I leaned against the wall.

"We think she has a large tumor," the doctor said, resting his index finger and forefinger in the area between his chest and throat. This could explain her lack of appetite and loss of weight.

"Now," using the wall for support, my father asked, "is it cancerous?"

With his eyes directly on my father, the doctor replied, "We think so."

My father then asked in a flat voice, "What's the bottom line?"

The doctor continued. "The earliest we could schedule her surgery is the day after tomorrow."

While I remained speechless, my father asked the tough question: "How long does she have?"

The doctor replied, "Probably three months."

Silently my father and I walked back to my mother's oppressive room. Her eyes were closed. I wanted to think this was her way of avoiding conversation and demonstrating some control. We let the nurse at the desk know we would return later. My father resigned himself to my driving him home that afternoon.

Nothing tried my patience more than standing on the lower step while my father attempted to unlock his back door. I had to discipline myself not to ask for his keys. The process of entering his house seemed endless to me. He started the search in his overcoat pockets, moved underneath to his sport coat pockets, then deeper, to his trouser pockets, and finally back to his overcoat pockets. Eventually he found the keys in his sport coat pocket. Which key was the house key? In the darkness of December, I watched his back while he at last inserted a key into the lock. I appreciated how important it was for him to be master. The door flew open. I was right behind him.

I observed how carefully and painstakingly he placed his coat on the hanger and hung it in the front hall closet. I realized the house would maintain its natural order while he was staying alone. My father always looked and dressed immaculately. He had very clean habits. When I was young he did the Sunday dishes following our traditional Sunday dinner. He would wipe the stainless-steel sink till it was free from any water spots. What I didn't expect was that each night of mother's hospital stay he would do his own laundry and hang it neatly on towel racks in the bathroom.

Suddenly, while walking back toward the kitchen, my father stopped short and turned to face me. "Listen carefully; I am only going to tell you this once. With your mother sick and in the hospital, I am alone. I will be looking for people to do for me. Janet, you be careful what you commit yourself to." I was touched but not surprised by his concern. As usual, he was one step ahead of me.

I stood in my mother's kitchen wondering what would come next. While my father's thoughts turned to Mother, my thoughts were focused on him. His forgetfulness and confusion concerned me the most. Although he left for work each morning at seven-thirty and returned at five o'clock, he was eighty-five years old. At work his sons-in-law and loyal employees watched over him. Here at home he would now be shuffling on his own. What if he tripped? Mother had a scatter rug between the dining room and kitchen. I didn't dare to remove it for fear my father would think I was taking over. I knew he was capable of using the stove but also capable of forgetting to turn it off. If I put something in the oven for him to warm up, he might fall asleep and, thinking he had already eaten, go off to bed. At this point I had no idea he had Alzheimer's disease. I simply thought of him as an aging parent. When he spoke I realized that he, too, was working a plan. "Gordon and Johnny work with me all day long and they don't need to come home at night to find me seated at their dinner tables. It is not the last meal I have at your house or your sister's that concerns me; it is the first."

I knew there was no changing his mind. I arranged his place setting at the kitchen table using a cloth napkin rather than the usual paper. Daddy needed something soft tonight. "I'm going home now to Gordon and the children," I said, "but I will be back with dinner all cooked and arranged on a plate at six o'clock."

A warm smile crossed his lips. "Great," he said. "I like your cooking."

It was three o'clock that December 1986 when I arrived home to make dinner for the family in a new way. Although I was alone in the house, I went straight to my bedroom and closed the door. I closed my eyes, inhaled deeply, and exhaled, allowing the tension from my head and shoulders to flow down my arms and out my fingertips. Quietly my body began to relax. I felt grateful I had taken a course in focusing and could use this technique as a tool. I chortled strangely to myself when I realized I had begun to plan my parents' dying process the way I planned a party.

Thoughts crowded in. My parents were courageous people who understood dying was as much a part of living as life itself. I knew they would not see themselves as victims. It was important to me I rise to their high standards, to take a positive attitude, to be responsible and organized, to take charge, not leave their dying process to chance. Try to see the whole picture. Family history told me I would be doing most of it. Would I suffer from burn-out? Where would anger fit in? I knew I would have to set boundaries.

Caring for Mother and my father would not be easy. I did not know if my commitment would last five days, five months, or as long as five years. I did not want to make myself sick. I knew to think, "balance." My natural instincts for long-range planning told me to do so. During these brief moments to myself, I resolved to continue my schooling and my part-time job at the Haverhill Girls Club. Two and a half days a week for myself and the rest of the time for my parents felt reasonable and responsible.

At forty I had returned to school and was currently studying expressive therapies at Lesley College in Cambridge, Massachusetts. I taught word processing and also directed an after-school program on self-esteem for girls age six to sixteen. As my mind wandered and I tried to organize a picture of the days ahead, I thought of my sister, Barbara, four years older than I, living across town and with her own concerns. Perhaps we should agree not to report to each other at the end of each day. I'd be too tired to talk. Besides, we would need that time for our families. I shouldn't forget to call Auntie Mae often. Mother had spoken to her sister every morning at nine-thirty for as long as I could remember. They would both miss the phone calls. My mind traveled to other practical matters. *Have I enough extra dishes to transport Daddy's dinner from my house? Remember to bring the picnic basket up from down in the cellar,* I thought. Suddenly I was petrified. How was I going to get him to let me make decisions and interact with the doctors? I resolved to build his trust.

I heard the back door open and my husband, Gordon, with his characteristic warmth, calling, "Hello." At first I feared he carried news of my mother's death. Then I realized it was close to dinner. The clock in the dining room struck five as I hung up the phone from talking to our daughter Cindy.

"I have an announcement to make," I said. Jeffrey and Valerie were standing impatiently waiting for a clearer explanation for what they had just overheard. Gordon was at the sink washing his hands. "As you heard, Grammie is in the hospital and Grampa is home doing who knows what. He refuses to come here for any meals or to stay overnight." They were hanging onto my every word, concern for me visible in their faces. I continued. "If during this time you are feeling left out or neglected, chances are you are. I don't want to sound harsh, but Grammie and Grampa need me and I want to be there for them. Here is your dinner. I am going to take this serving to Grampa because he's too confused to use the stove and refuses to have a housekeeper. Believe it or not, he doesn't want the neighbors to think he's living with another woman while Grammie's in the hospital." Laughter cleared the air.

I passionately wanted my children to know how to take care of themselves, even at an early age, so that one day they would be able to make their own decisions, form their own relationships, and have their own lives. At sixteen I had given each an alarm clock and a calendar because I wanted to encourage them to be in charge of themselves. Once they obtained their own driver's licenses, they set up their own appointments and drove themselves in and out of the city. I made sure they were competent navigators into the bigger world. When they were in elementary and high school I developed headaches that lasted eleven to twenty-one days out of a month and were several notches above severe; my headaches also inspired me to encourage the children to take care of themselves. I was either controlled in denial ("I'm fine; my head is burning up inside, but I'm fine") or else in a pain-free euphoria. My behavior oftentimes excluded the beautiful middle ground where there is warm serenity. I have since developed more perspective on my parents, the whole stressful independent way they treated me, and how in many ways I was recovering from my own upbringing. I required to be an independent person, more than most. Both my parents, for very different reasons, were forced to leave their houses at an early age. Hence they could not give me support they had not received when they were growing up. In a matter-of-fact way they had insisted I make the major decisions for myself. This presented tremendous challenges for a young girl. I was sent away to summer camp from the time I was six years old. Neither of my parents had learned how to swim or be carefree to play. They were eager for me to learn. My security came less from affection than from a sense of order, dignity, control, success, purpose, and all the details of daily life that were inscribed in a sense of strength and reliability.

My children always had their own independent relationship with their grandparents, and I encouraged that. When they were visiting either grandparent it was not uncommon for them to bring along friends. During the elementary school years they oftentimes rode their bicycles up to Eastland Terrace and shared homemade chocolate chip cookies, ginger ale, fun and lively conversation with my mother. Once they had their driver's licenses they would cruise down to the dealership and visit with their grandfather at work. "I remember asking him about

automobiles and sales, but he never wanted to discuss it."
Valerie says. "He was more interested to know what we
were learning in school and he liked to talk politics. He
would often play the devil's advocate to encourage us to
consider new ideas. I never left my grandfather's presence, even when he was in the Alzheimer's unit, without
suspecting he was still consciously teaching me to think."

My parents loved seeing their grandchildren. Their
presence awakened in my mother some of the happier
times in her childhood; as "one of the kids" she offered a
good ear without judgment. Together they created a circle
of happy youthful safety. My father especially derived
great pleasure from his carefree, secure grandchildren
because his own childhood had been cut short abruptly
when his father died at eleven and he had gone to work.

My father was always fascinated by other people who
came from large families and worked very hard. Eleanor,
my mother's hairdresser, came one day to comb my
mother's hair for a special occasion. She and my father
got to talking. She said how she was from a family of
twelve. "Tell me," he said: "How in the world do people
bring up so many children?"

Eleanor explained how her father bought eight double loaves of bread a day and had thirty quarts of milk delivered every other day. "My father got up each morning
between five and five-thirty went to the east window, and
prayed thanks." Eleanor continued, "Each morning he
made a canning kettle full of oatmeal. We had that for
breakfast with a loaf of Italian bread he had hidden from
the day before. We never went hungry."

"I can't imagine what that was like. I didn't have a
brother, and I didn't have a sister. It would have been
nice."

Eleanor replied, "You're lucky; your mother probably doted on you. I have to get back to work now."

With a twinkle in his eye, he said, "Don't leave. Comb her hair over again, maybe on the other side. I haven't had such a good afternoon in a long time."

Driving in the dark streets with the picnic basket on the floor next to me, I was reminded of my childhood Halloween night in my Little Red Riding Hood costume. I could use my own key to enter the house, but what if I frightened Daddy to death? *No,* I thought, *I will stand here and ring the bell two more times. By then if he doesn't answer I will go down the street and call him from a pay phone. Maybe he has fallen asleep.* Another three rings and I heard him fumbling with the lock. Here we go again! With a big grin on his face he opened the storm door and graciously welcomed me in. The place setting I had arranged earlier was no longer there. He noticed my hesitation and said "I'll eat in the den and watch the news at the same time. I don't want to sit next to your mother's empty chair. And by the way, I couldn't hear the doorbell very well with the television going. Tomorrow I'll have the electrician come and connect the back doorbell to a bell here in the den."

Still carrying the basket, I followed him into the den. I thought to myself, *One moment he's pale and grieving and the next he's organizing the house with his characteristic authority and expertise.*

He lowered himself into his chair and positioned the TV table in front of him. Eating here was a new experience for him. "This feels nice," he said, rubbing his thumb and index finger along the edges of the napkin as he lowered it onto his lap. "You go home now. This meal looks delicious and I don't want it to get cold."

I felt the resentment building shortly after I awoke the next morning. Everyone else in the family had visited Mother yesterday, while my time had been spent with my father. What if she died in surgery? What if I never got my turn to visit? I knew in my heart I would never forgive the other family members.

At 6:30 A.M. I pulled into the hospital parking lot. I had never been in a hospital at that hour of day. I walked with authority and intention.

The elevator was empty. Leaning against the metal wall, I felt the railing pressed securely against my lower back. I went about calming myself. When the elevator stopped I took one giant step into the hallway and saw the familiar figure of my father just inside the doorway of my mother's room. Quickly I jumped back into the elevator before the door had a chance to close. I should have known. What would ever make me think I could be one step ahead of this man? Returning to the parking lot, I moved my car two rows back and to the left behind his. I sat and waited for him to leave. I waited patiently, feeling my resentment build while at the same time I longed to remain reasonable. During my adult years my mother and I had been enjoying each other. I wanted to share one last laugh and twinkle of the eye with her before she disappeared into the good night. The minute I saw him get into his car and drive away I was back on the elevator and entering room 303. Maybe it was the morning sun bringing hope into the room or the stillness of my mother lying quietly against the freshly pressed sheets with the traditional tucked corners. Her delicate soft smile, the way she arched her eyebrows, expressed her surprise and her joy in seeing me. We were alone. Our eyes held a calming devotion. They spoke volumes. Holding my mother's hand, I told her what I thought she wanted to hear: "Daddy's fine, Mother. He is fine." Then the orderlies came.

Standing in front of the elevator door, I remembered Victor Frankel's words in *Man's Search for Meaning:* "When all the familiar goals in life are snatched away, what alone remains is the ability to choose one's attitude."

I stopped to telephone Gordon on the lobby phone on my way back to the parking lot. He said that my father was at work and was planning on staying there while my mother was in surgery. My sister, Barbara, and I waited in our respective homes. I began to rely on Gordon in a new way.

My father received the phone call first. Mother's surgery had produced gallstones rather than a cancerous tumor. We were all exhilarated. Sitting across from my father and Dr. Goldbaum, I listened and watched intensely as the surgeon sketched the procedure where he removed the stones. He was confident that her appetite would soon increase. Watching this successful surgeon's pleasure and enthusiasm toward his work transcended my uncertainty. Dr. Goldbaum talked about the benefits of being thin when undergoing surgery and how with Mother weighing less than seventy-five pounds he was able to "get in and out quickly," resulting in her having less anesthesia, which in turn made the process of surgery less threatening. My head was overflowing with thoughts of celebration when I telephoned our local florist and asked to have a giant poinsettia delivered to the surgeon's office. I was feeling excited and giddy. "The largest one you have," I added. I signed the card: "Beautiful People cause Beautiful Things to Happen. Thank you, The Marble Family." My father was overjoyed when I told him

I had the bill for the flowers sent to him. "Good; that's one bill I feel privileged to pay."

Dr. Munter never referred to the misdiagnosis, and I was glad. You can be certain my father never complained. We got what we prayed for. I could not spend my time or energies scrutinizing the doctor. Due to malnutrition and respiratory complications my mother remained in the hospital nine weeks. During that time I developed a more insightful and sophisticated slant toward medical professionals. I saw how hard they worked. I was impressed that they avoided using my mother's age for rationalization. Yet when I heard Dr. Munter say, "I'm going skiing this Wednesday afternoon and an associate will be in charge of your mother," I panicked! I remember wondering if Dr. Munter ever thought of my mother while he was on the ski slopes. I grew to hope he didn't. The more I learned to understand the importance of balance in my own life, the more I was able to appreciate doctors and how they dealt with the discipline of creating balance in their own lives.

My father went directly to Mother's room while I phoned Gordon and Barbara, reiterating Dr. Goldbaum's detailed analysis of the surgery. When I returned to the third floor and room 303, my eyes moved between my father seated and Mother lying in bed with her eyes closed. Tubes were everywhere. I saw flashing numbers on unfamiliar instruments. Being unable to interpret what I was looking at frightened me the most. My father looked like a fifth-grader sitting in a first-grader's chair, his upper torso bent forward with his elbows resting on his legs and his forehead cupped in the palm of his hands. The scene made my mind spin while my body remained motionless. My heart wanted to reach out, but it just wept. The two of them looked so lost.

"Daddy, I'm going downstairs to the lobby to use the pay phone. I'm getting some private duty nurses in here. We'll have them around-the-clock for three days, and then we'll evaluate the situation.". My father never had the experience of people taking charge of his life. He never had allowed it. This was the beginning of a new era.

I had been spunky from an early age. In high school I took my father's attitude toward community; I was involved in student government and knew how to have a voice. I attended city council meetings each Tuesday evening with my friend Marilyn. Our history teacher handed over the third-period history class for us to run each Wednesday. My parents wanted to send me to private school. I took the situation into my own hands by telephoning the admissions office to say that they had come into financial difficulties. I hid the acceptance letter in my pink hanky box until I felt sure the position had been filled. When I told my parents at the dinner table my father applauded my behavior by saying, "Looks as though you know what you want. You went through a lot not to go there." Mother chorused, "Jesus, Mary, and Joseph, where did she come from?"

I pulled out the thick yellow page phone book and looked under "Nursing Services." I was too rattled to stay with the fine print so went directly to the largest ad. Mother's frail figure lying in bed kept flashing before my eyes, but not nearly as clearly as my father's expression of bewilderment. Whoever was going to care for Mother would also be dealing with my father. We needed to have someone with a intuitive nature and an abundance of common sense. I requested RNs, presuming they would have more experience and maturity. Elizabeth Carey was the first nurse to arrive. Looking back, I believe she was a direct gift from God. A former nun, she brought God and prayer back into my parents' life. For this I will be eternally grateful.

My parents came from very different religious backgrounds. My mother was raised in a Catholic middle-class family. Her father had been a bricklayer, and her mother a housewife. To look at my mother you would never have thought she sang solo at the St. James Church when age thirteen. Her petite body didn't look as though it had enough volume. She had four brothers and five sisters. When my mother married my father she was excommunicated. My father was an only child. His father died when he was only eleven years old, and thus he was unable, like three generations that preceded him, to attend Dartmouth College. As he was a stoic self-made businessman, I oftentimes heard him say with strict Protestant ethic, "People don't give up on their cars, why would they give up on life?"

I especially wanted my father to know the apple had not fallen far from the tree, for I knew that gaining my father's trust would be my greatest hurdle. I sensed one day that now was my opportunity to show my father what I had learned from him; his strengths could now manifest through me. My father respected smart, self-made, forceful people. I sighted examples of his character in me. "Daddy," I heard myself saying, "with my brains and your experience we can do anything."

My mother's recovery was clearly taking its toll on my father. In the fifth week of Mother's hospital stay, standing by his back door resigned to his weariness, he said, "Janet, you do good work. Tomorrow you speak to the doctor and let me know what he says." I knew then that I had earned his trust. In those days I only allowed

25

myself tears when something had been resolved. As I backed out his driveway, the tears of relief and pride flowed freely.

Dr. Munter, reported that although Mother was suffering from malnutrition and respiratory disorder her prognosis was good. He believed that the scar on her lung had possibly been there from as far back as her early childhood and that the injured tissue suggested she had suffered undiagnosed tuberculosis as a child. "This tells me your mother is a strong-willed woman with powerful healing capabilities, and an innate desire to live," he said.

On January 20 Mother was in the intensive care unit and on a respirator for the third time. She continued to grab fiercely at the tubing, determined to remove it from her breathing passage. The nurses believe this was her way of telling people she wanted to die. Concerned this might be so and anxious to meet my mother's every desire, I related this interpretation to Dr. Munter. With a hint of frustration he sounded off. "If your mother wanted to die she has had plenty of opportunities before now," he said. "She is simply telling us to take the respirator out so that she can breathe on her own and the added oxygen is getting in her way. I will have the nurses start weaning her tomorrow." On January 23 my mother was breathing on her own. With joyful childlikeness the nurses referred to her as a living miracle.

In my anxiety, however, my imagination ran rampant. I developed an uncontrollable need to know in advance what I would find at the hospital. As the elevator rose so did my heightened anticipation. I would stop first at the nurses' station to check and double-check on my mother's condition. I judged the nurses by their attention, as I let myself be taught by them the nature and language of her illness. I had an attentive ear and a good memory. I would remove my eyeglasses, hoping to appear more powerful and be more clearly understood. I interrogated, "How are her vital signs? Has the doctor been in and did he make changes regarding her medication? Her breathing, which was giving her great difficulty yesterday, how is it today?" I'd start down the corridor walking quickly and feeling full of myself, like a charge nurse who loves her job and is good at it. In this way I worked up my courage again and again to see Mother. When I neared her room I would stop short and change my pace to baby steps, hoping someone might call out, "Red light," sending me back to start. The old walnut hospital door loomed huge and awesome, slightly opened. I leaned, angling my head every which way to get a peek at her. If the report at the desk had been bad, I felt relieved when I saw she was either sleeping or resting with her eyes closed. I had given myself permission to leave if what I saw frightened me too much.

I remember when I was a child my father telling me to "wait and see" what is going on inside a room before you enter talking. Standing silently in the doorway, I would face Mother and her daily chart hanging like a bad threat from the footboard. I made a habit of observing myself through her eyes. I'd give myself what I called spot checks before entering her room. I did not want her to see me looking tense and frazzled. I composed my face, like putting on makeup, throwing my shoulders back and intentionally lowering them into a more relaxed position. I would take one last pause, enough to orientate myself to her fragile condition. I did not want to make her nervous and overly curious about me, nor did I want to bring her germs. I kept a careful distance between us. I carried my kisses in my heart.

Mother's position in her bed determined where it

27

would be most comfortable for her to view me. Her eyes gave me direction as to where I should stand. During the crucial times when she was most weak and lying flat on her back, I leaned on the edge of the bed rails. The cool sensation from the steel bars helped to keep me focused. She had thick gray hair, which added fullness to her drawn face. Her teeth had been capped a dozen years back, leaving her cheeks in their natural shape. Her recent loss of weight created a more distinct ripple effect under her cheekbones, slightly above her jaw. It wasn't until I looked at her arms, thin and peppered with bruises brought about by the needles, that my stomach turned. I had to fight not to lower my eyes. Mother already had been self-conscious about her spindly arms long before she entered the hospital. It was for that reason she had worn long-sleeved dresses in the summer, unless, of course, she was home alone and it was hot and humid outside. I would exaggerate the words and enunciate clearly, "Mother, it is important to me and to your recovery. You understand perfectly that you do not have a disease. You have what Daddy and now I call 'mechanical problems.' As soon as the doctors figure it out you will be fine."

She would glare softly. "I know!"

Because I felt Mother's skin was being violated all day long I seldom touched its thin tissue. When she was well enough to sit up, I would stand at the foot of her bed, where we could talk without her having to turn her head. I would softly cup my hand over the top of her covered toes and sometimes squeezed them gently. The feel of the white tennis peds I had bought for her made me warm and cozy. I liked to think the warmth of my body soothed her. When she was seated in the hospital chair with a pillow puffed and tucked behind her head, I would sit at her feet on a stool I found under her bed. Sometimes as we spoke together I traced with my fingertips along the folds of thin white blanket lying across her lap covering her petite, bony kneecaps, no bigger than toddler fists. As I talked she would nod off to sleep.

Slowly I became accustomed to the details of hospital life. I was pleasantly surprised the day I entered Mother's room and no longer felt chilled and intimidated by the digital monitor machine, the chrome stand that held her intravenous feeding bags, nor by the clear green oxygen cup that hung on the wall. I saw them for what they were and was reassured by their presence. I was careful never to ask Mother how she was feeling, because she was compelled as a patient to be a hostess, I realized how challenging it was for her to be courteous to all of us who wanted to be helpful.

Mother was taking charge of her recovery by receiving only what benefited her. There were days she did not have the energy to deal with my desire to help her and she pretended to be asleep. I had seen her do this many times to my father, but never did I expect her to do this to me. My feelings were hard to deal with. I experienced rejection. Then one day I figured it out. Mother was in the midst of shutting herself down and letting her body heal itself. She had not been turning me away, as I perceived it, she had been turning me off. She wasn't talking about inner healing; she was doing it. While she appeared frail and weak, she was cultivating an inner strength.

It was not only at the hospital with Mother I had feelings of rejection; I oftentimes felt let down by my friends, except for my most intimate ones. I handled my feelings of disappointment by walking around with a tight upper lip. While other members of the family were receiving phone calls of concern and sympathy, my telephone remained relatively silent. People knew I was busy during the day running back and forth to the hospital and to my father with his nightly meals. I suspected that few people would want to hear my nervously detailed health reports, yet I wanted more compassion. I felt no shame in asking people for what I thought my parents needed. Admiring cards gave my father a pleasant distraction while he was visiting Mother. Her respiratory condition caused us to discourage flowers.

Over many years I had become adept at projecting a positive attitude. When I met people who asked how my mother was "coming along," to protect myself I jubilated in her fighting spirit.

To protect myself and because in my family there was much denial of feelings, for many years I kept my headaches a secret. I hid them from everyone until after many days of unremitting pain sometimes I would break down in tears and tell Gordon. Conscientious to a fault, if anything went wrong I thought that I was responsible. So I gave the impression I was an exceptionally happy, positive person. Exacerbated by my need to keep them hidden, sometimes the pain was so intense that I would sit on my hands to keep from opening the door and throwing myself out of the car. I would kneel on my bed pillow with both hands clenched to the headboard, knocking my head against the wall to change the pattern of the pain. Even though headaches caused me struggles and suffering, I learned, as I fought feverishly to stay oriented, to use that focused energy in a positive, productive way.

When I was young our family didn't run to doctors, I didn't see medicine tablets around the house. When feeling irritated my mother cleaned and tore closets apart and my father played cards or another round of golf. While I was caring for my parents I nevertheless had a series of relationships with health professionals. I lost trust in a well-known headache specialist when he increased my prescriptions through the mail. I wasn't as angry as I was sad. I confronted him. Because it scared the living daylights out of me that the doctor would be that irresponsible. I developed a healthy, stubborn obsession with purity. I wouldn't even take an aspirin, but just accepted the pain. Although my mother took Haley's Headache Powder, I didn't even want to take that.

Soon I was visiting a chiropractor biweekly. My twenty-minute twice-a-week appointment was a successful alternative to drugs. Dr. Fowler Jr. was a young man who had a knack for finding the soul's dislocations. I realized that he was a mentor to me quite early on in the relationship, and I was hungry for the guidance he had to give. He reminded me of my father, though a much younger man. He carried authority, knowledge, and wisdom. I liked his style of teaching. He was quick and abrupt, like my father. Although I didn't hesitate to throw out some of what he preached, I paid fierce attention and did not forget a word he said. He was not just helping me on the physical level but was also offering me some real guidance and inspiration. It was because of him that I started turning around some of my negative thinking. One day he said, "If I were you I would take a Dale Carnegie course and read Norman Vincent Peale's *Power of Positive Thinking*."

Positive thinking taught me I could make a difference, and when I could make a difference and didn't I was not only disappointed in myself; I felt I was not living up to my own potential. Even though I didn't have a traditional job, I had my own job description, which required me to live up to my own expectations. What better way for me to show God my appreciation of His gift of life?

Being imaginative and open to new ideas was my salvation. As I was determined to be resilient, my headaches became my motivations for new learning. On my own I studied the theory of chiropractic; I wanted to understand the fundamental procedure before placing the alignment of my body in the hands of another person. Also, I thought that being knowledgeable about my treatment, I could in some way improve the outcome. Researching chiropractic whetted my appetite for other studies to raise my level of consciousness.

While taking a course in ethics I wrote a term paper on animal abuse. When I read how the average American by his seventieth birthday will have eaten 14 steers, 1,050 chickens, 3.5 lambs, and 25.2 hogs, I gave up meat. When the course was over I returned to eating meat, but only on occasion and with a new sense of awareness. I also took several courses in philosophy. I learned to break down a situation and look at it from various viewpoints in order to make a moral decision, seeing happiness as an intrinsic good. I liked this utilitarian approach, maximizing the greatest amount of happiness for the greatest amount of people. I also saw my own happiness had no more value than anyone else's. These became the questions I asked myself when I was problem-solving with the nurses and my parents. There were times I was attracted to a course simply by the title. I remember taking a psychology course simply because in the descriptive text it mentioned "Searching for Self-Fulfillment in a world Turned Upside Down." I took a course in movement therapy and was challenged to put emotions to movement. When my whole body was burning and I was unable to distinguish one muscle from another, I would play soft music, get down on the floor, and move the same way I imagined myself as having moved when I was a baby.

Once I learned how to move I went on and took classes on how to be still. I studied first *The Religions of Man,* by Huston Smith, then areas of meditation.

When my mother was ill I took particular notice of my dreams. In my early childhood I had sometimes been very disturbed by my dreams. Now I began to record my current dreams, which moved me to the works of Carl Jung and his dream theories. I am definitely not what I would think of as a scholar. Yet I was a closet feminist in those days and more liberal than other members of my family. So when I found myself at the Carl Jung Institute in Boston, seated at a small, round table in the library with six very accomplished scholars, all graduates of the Carl Jung Institute in Switzerland, studying the women in Carl Jung's life, I knew I'd gone too far. I continued to show up for the full eight weeks of the course.

I learned that my unconscious had the ability to un-ravel stressful, complicated issues, and I discovered new ways to rise above pain through "active imagination." One day when my headache absorbed my attention I imagined miniature astronauts wearing small tanks on their backs, vacuuming, washing down, and lubricating the pain inside my head. I couldn't deny how effectively creative I could be when "out of my mind" with pain. I learned to live more in the present moment, to be less re-stricted by my personal history, and to turn my future over to God. Freedom to create my life through God's will was what I was now seeking. As I look back on my behav-ior I am surprised at how spunky and persevering I was.

I became more aware of myself in relationship with nature. I grew a new respect for nature: When Gordon went to protect the bird feeder from the squirrels I saw how the little creatures would outsmart him every time. I took to studying the patterns of the lead birds that flocked overhead, identifying with the leader.

Back then it was not uncommon for me to stop by the side of the road for five or ten minutes to watch bulldozers hard at work. One night after dinner my husband took me to John Deere. I climbed on all the tractors, and pretended I was driving. Gordon had a good sense of humor about it; he didn't say, "Look at my peculiar wife." Full of Taurus energies, I wanted to experience working with nature in a powerful way.

My instincts told me to bring Mother everything that would comfort her during her hospital stay. Using her recipes, I prepared for her daily tasty meals served on her everyday dinnerware. I delivered them promptly, in the picnic basket at mealtime. I overdid one day when I gave her a frilly Valentine napkin.

Mother's increased awareness brought with it concern for my father's sadness. For his sake I wanted her to look healthier. I began by purchasing a soft pink satin long-sleeved night gown with tiny rosebuds floating across the top. I contacted Sadie, mother's former dressmaker, and asked if she would open the nightgown up the back with Velcro closures. The following day when my father telephoned, I heard his smile of relief: "I think your mother is coming around. She was all dolled up in a fancy gown today, and I've heard people say that's a good sign."

Whenever I didn't know what to do I prayed. I prayed on elevators and in parking lots, on street corners, and simply driving along. I prayed knowingly and unknowingly. It became my daily chant. With my right hand tightly fisted I would push up and down on the weight of the world repeating, "I can do all things through Christ who strengtheneth me" (Philippians 4:13). To avoid sleepless nights, upon waking I immediately went into prayer. Truly, if I awakened on an inhale I was in prayer on the exhale. I had a nighttime mantra as well. "Dear God, please give my mother the courage and strength to face whatever You have planned for her. And please also fill my father's heart with peace and tranquillity."

I learned control from my father, and now he was starting to show raw emotion I had never seen before. It was Thursday morning, February 12, nine weeks since my mother's admission to the hospital. I was at my parents' home checking last-minute details before Mother returned from the hospital. The French doors swung open; I stood inside the sun-filled family room smiling, feeling satisfied. I had accomplished what I set out to do. Mother's comfort and needs had been met with minimal disturbance of my father's comfort zone. I put the rose puff over the commode so my father wouldn't see it. The hospital bed was placed in the corner of the room with two large picture windows on each outside wall, a perfect location for watching Mother Nature perform her miracles. I was feeling full of myself. I was the daughter of a walking miracle and bursting with pride.

My father's voice came from behind out of nowhere. Before I knew it he was standing next to me. "Get all that stuff out of here," he said. Pointing to the puff, he continued. "Get that thing out of here, too. I will be taking care of your mother myself."

The words came straight from my belly calmly and clearly as I responded, "You look here, Daddy. I am fifty years of age and this time I am calling the shots. You cannot take care of Mother because she needs more than what you have to offer, and furthermore, nurses will be here twenty-four hours a day until Mother can do for herself. I am your daughter; I know what I am doing. Now, sit in that blue chair over there and be quiet."

Within moments the hospital van rounded the corner. My father held the storm door open while a nurse pushed the wheelchair and Mother into the living room. All sixty three pounds of her sat high and mighty, wearing her familiar camel hair coat. A blue print scarf hanging loosely around her neck added color and fullness to her tired face. As she was wheeled into the family room she lowered her head and sobbed with relief. The nurse crouched down next to her and held her hand quietly. Their heads rested against each other as they exchanged whispers. The expressions of tenderness moved me quietly to the back hall landing, where alone I shed my own welcome home tears.

2

Be bold, and mighty forces will come to your aid.
—Basil King

This day like many other days I heard myself mumbling, "Give until it feels good."

All the time my mother was ill in the hospital my father's symptoms were submerged. When she came home and started to recover we were dismayed to see him, a man who had been so highly disciplined all his life, sometimes totally out of control. We noticed more his primal feelings, especially jealousy and rage. At the end of his workday his angry behavior began to manifest the moment he walked through the back door. I understood that seeing my mother weak and dependent caused him intense anxiety. We hid the scales on which we weighed Mother every morning hoping she had gained some weight and also the walker and nursing commode from his view. We tried to keep the house looking as normal as possible.

Mother believed if she looked alert he might be less apt to criticize her. The nurses supported her in this. When he came home every morning at 10:30, Mother was always dressed to greet him even if she was planning a lazy day. She napped during the afternoon, in order to keep my father company at night, and only before retiring would she change into her sleepwear.

My father's daytime devotion was endearing, but his nighttime ritual was cruel. He would fervently interrogate my mother as to her food intake for the day, how far and for how long she had walked, and if she had used the walker or attempted to use the cane. His interrogations took on a tone of desperation, and we wanted to minimize this criticism and bullying. Mother's great motivation for recovering was that he needed her.

My mother attempted to diffuse his rage by ignoring his outbursts, I tried to compensate for it by visiting her several times a day. The nurses knew to leave the back door unlocked and ajar for my dramatic arrivals. Like a supply train hooting in with a goodly supply of eagerness and positive energy, I would greet my mother and the nurses with grand jubilation. Looking back on it now, I can imagine at times they must have cringed at my steam engine approach. From the beginning of the six years of my life with my parents' dying process I considered it my personal victory to bring humor and laughter into my parents' house. They each required positive reinforcement due to the stress of the other's condition. I saw myself as that strengthening force. All my visits were intense. I felt I needed to take total responsibility for bringing lighthearted, effervescent moments into my mother's life. Yet I would often sit at the opposite end of the room, fearful I might be carrying germs. In grade school I had been labeled "chatty." Now my nervous chatter took a new course. I was always careful to begin slowly, letting Mother express whatever was on her mind. I watched for the expression in her eyes and my own intuition. She was full of gumption and had a wonderful sense of humor. Sometimes her smile told me she was ready for a good belly laugh.

Living with my father's unpredictability caused everyone uneasiness. Mother required a lot of attention, and while she and the nurses were developing a rapport, my father was feeling left out. His mood swings caused Mother and the nurses to communicate differently when he was at home. Their laughter was less hearty, and they guarded themselves. My father had always been a stickler about teasing and gossip. My visits were also different when my father was at home. One day I noticed, much to my surprise, that my father was showing signs of jealousy because my mother was getting well. Unconsciously he saw her as a rival for attention.

My mother's behavior toward her husband became increasingly dry and cold. Her techniques hadn't changed over the years. She used either the silent treatment or the proverbial stare that told us something was wrong, but we were not to talk about it. I had the luxury of distancing myself; she lived with his increasingly raw outbursts. When our home telephone rang in the middle of the night I simply told myself, "I can't handle it." My dear husband, Gordon, who had quietly and skillfully long been the family's helpmate, took over where my emotional strength gave out. God bless him, he was willing. We strove to keep my parents together, a family unit, as well as a household unit. Nevertheless, I felt my sister, Barbara, and I needed to take primary responsibility during that year when Mother was fighting to get up on her feet and my father's confusion and irritability was accelerating. Mother never recuperated to the point where she would have been able to take care of him. Because his needs kept growing, we soon realized that we would require the help of nurses. We did not see a nursing home as an option as long as my father still had his money available to himself. Rather than have a housekeeper who would be there all the time, we made the decision to have a variety of nurses. With their varied personalities, they were a catalyst that helped to make my parents' home a busy world of its own. I saw with increasing clarity that if money couldn't return my parents to good health, it could buy options. My father's money was buying choices relating to their death process. Our intention was not to pamper Mother but to treat her in the manner to which she was accustomed, maintaining her life with dignity. I knew the nurses were a luxury and that we had a privileged life. My parents had never talked about spending or saving money. Money was not a topic of discussion any more than someone being in "the family way" would be. As a child I saw the *Wall Street Journal* in the house, but I never realized it was serving a purpose.

I often heard the nurses comment on the devotion my mother had to her family and that my father had to the community. His family ethic trickled all the way down through the grandchildren. Over the years, when coming home from college for school breaks and holidays, they had established a routine. No sooner did they walk through the back door, throw their duffel bags down in the back hall, and run upstairs to check things out and return to the kitchen than they would announce, "I'm going to drive up and see Grammie and Grampa." They always knew they would be warmly received. My mother had a way of inspiring her grandchildren across the generations. "We may not see the world the same way, I accept that, and I still love you and myself" was her general attitude. Our children had always taken pleasure in visiting their grandparents.

In June of 1987 the lawn man was mowing the lawn when my father pulled into the driveway home from work, earlier than usual. The young man followed him to the back door. With sincere warmth my father invited him into the house. "What can I do for you?" my father asked, who was often exceptionally nice to strangers.

"My name is Kevin Ingalls. My father was Louis Ingalls." The young man continued on. "When I was a child my father spoke of you often. He enjoyed telling the story of you inviting him into your office one day while he waited for his car to be repaired. You asked him how things were, and Dad explained about his six-week-old son's weakening kidneys and how they didn't expect the infant to live. Mr. Marble, that is when you told Dad about a Boston specialist and set up an appointment for my parents to meet with him. I am that six-week-old boy, and I want to thank you for saving my life."

Raising his right arm and waving his hand in a downward motion, my father replied, "Oh hell, back then I did that sort of thing all the time."

Now, at eighty six years of age, before he had been diagnosed with Alzheimer's disease, my father was still leaving the house at 7:30 A.M. and driving himself to work one mile away. Nurses and outsiders were hounding the family to have his driver's license taken away. Even at his worst he had no difficulty navigating his own narrow driveway and garage, yet the moment my father left the house Beth called the dealership and the family surveillance team went into action. They hid behind snowbanks and around corners and patiently waited for my father to exit E-Z Way cleaners with his laundered shirts. My father had been a good citizen, never asked society for favors in return; he had taken responsibility for himself his entire life. He wasn't about to back down on the issue of losing his license without a good fight. Neither was I.

I sensed my chances were better with our clergyman

than a doctor. Through my thirty-year commitment to the Girls Club I saw myself as an advocate for young girls; now I was developing a new consciousness toward the elderly. I set out to find the answer I wanted to hear. "Tell me, Frank," I asked, "because you are a minister, you probably interact with as many elderly as anyone does. Just because people aren't comfortable with my father's driving, do we really need to take his license away? Can't we bend the rules a little? There are young people driving around with their legs hanging out the car window while their hands beat on the steering wheel to the sound of the stereo. Let's not forget driving drunken drivers. My father only travels one route from his house to his dealership and from the car dealership home. He has never wandered from his routine. Besides, God seems to take care of the elderly in traffic, and we know that He is good creating order."

Frank straightened himself in his chair; I focused on my breathing. "Janet, with the speed at which I see your father driving, whoever he hit wouldn't fall down."

The next time someone questioned my father's driving I simply smiled and said, "We spoke to our clergyman and he says it is fine."

We were custodians of the dying process, striving to emulate the spirit in which my parents had lived. With our families' financial resources we turned the household into a private nursing home with nurses and nurses' stations. My parents were no strangers to having a person live in their house. Years back Doja had lived with them for ten years. The nurses and my parents had already become familiar with one another while Mother was in the hospital. What they needed now was a new set of ground rules. The nurses were asked by my parents not to wear uniforms, although they could wear white to feel profes-

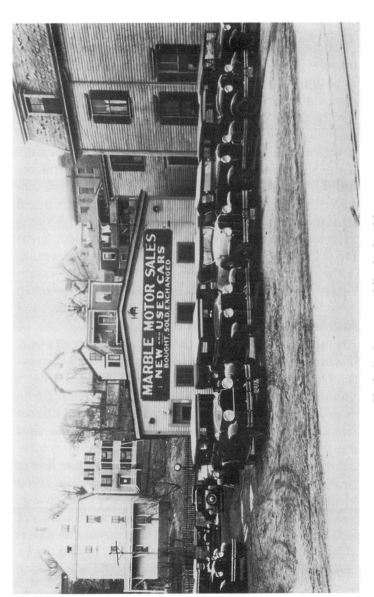

My father's automobile dealership

sional. It was not unusual for my father to comment on how nice they looked in bright colors. After a while the nurses, as is typical of women, started dressing for my father. It was another indication to me we were achieving lightness within the household. The nurses had their meals with my parents. They could see how conversation and stimulation was good for my father as well as Mother. They were never referred to as nurses in front of my father, only by name, or as "the girls"; otherwise, even if his mind was clear, he would have responded by asking, "Who's sick?" After a while the nurses felt comfortable using the telephone; I sometimes felt "the girls" were embarrassed, and preferred not to receive calls. One nurse brought mending for the early-evening hours. Mother would get a kick out of seeing the latest in adolescent fashion. The more regard the nurses were given, the more freely they voiced their concerns to one another. The result eventually was a tightly knit network of helpers. In this swirl the household relaxed with storytelling and laughter that penetrated even to the kitchen.

My father defined people in terms of their work ethic. You'd hear him say, "He's a hard worker," or, "He's a person who gives you your money's worth." That is why it was important we had people on Eastland Terrace who did their job well. We consistently had wonderful nurses and did not want to make any unexpected changes that could interrupt the flow. The main objective was to have continuity, even if this meant from time to time we had to pick up the slack ourselves when nursing services failed us. According to the contract, my parents' situation was to have a monthly evaluation. When I saw this did not happen I paid closer attention and appraised the situation. I had to make a decision to transform my anxieties into positive energy.

For a private and independent person like my mother to turn her house over to total strangers was a major challenge. Mother was from the era of bread and butter plates and fish on Friday. "These modern girls do things differently," she'd say. There was never any question that Mother was still in charge of her household, even though for her to organize her thoughts was now a struggle. The nurses were sensitive regarding her limitations and her feelings of disconnectedness. She was still too weak to stand alone. Beth would sit her in front of the refrigerator while she told them what foods to discard and what ones to add to the grocery order. Previously Mother's refrigerator had been trim, like she was, with no extra bulk, but now with the number of people in the house eating throughout the day, my mother was buying unusual quantities, one clear indication of how her house didn't seem the same to her anymore. In the late afternoons she and the nurse would move into the kitchen. Mother would settle into her rocking chair next to the hall landing and take on the role of a cooking instructor. The nurses were eager to learn and even try out new recipes on their families. Every Thursday morning the food order was phoned in. Unable to do the work, at least Mother could feel that she had participated.

I had never heard my mother complain, "Why me?" though there were days, particularly in the beginning, when she felt raw frustration. A woman who had never stayed in bed after seven and had always been dressed before breakfast was now welcoming family visitors, late morning, dressed in her pale pink quilted robe with matching pink slippers. Too weak to walk alone, she would sit in the family room, her eyes looking straight ahead out the front windows. If the window shades with matching tassels were hanging unevenly, she tried not to complain. The "young girls" had enough to do with taking care of her, learning the ropes, and attending to my father. How could she bother them with something as simple as straightening out a shade? I tried to predict what she would want ahead of time.

I had had previous experience in being dutiful, accepting responsibility, and learning to be conscious of my parents' health. In late June of 1957, when my family was living at our summer house in Rye Beach, New Hampshire, twenty-five miles from Haverhill, I was taking a summer course in politics and public opinion at the University of New Hampshire. The day had been hot and humid, but my father had played his regular weekend round of golf. Because of the heat I must have been sleeping lightly when I heard my mother call to come quickly. I saw my father sitting on the side of his twin bed, fright in his eyes and perspiration pouring down his face. On his lap was a hand towel Mother had given him so he could wipe his brow. I was not accustomed to seeing my father fearful and out of control. My father asked her to call his longtime friend and physician Dr. Consentino. They were relieved when the doctor offered to make a house call. They were outright stunned when he told Mother to find herself another bed. He had decided to spend the night and "keep an eye on Ted's condition." I remember the doctor waving her out the door when she wanted to put fresh sheets on her bed. By the following morning he diagnosed my father's heart attack.

Afterward my father made significant changes in his life. Whatever the doctor suggested he did half that amount. If he was told to walk one mile, he would walk a half-mile instead. He was told not to raise his arms above his head, so he sat with them folded in his lap. They told him not to participate in stressful games of gin rummy, so he gave up his Tuesday night card group. It was the first time in his life he walked away from confrontation, even if it was an irritated customer at his business. When my father was released from the hospital I was the one expected to be his daily companion. My mother did not drive, it was summertime, I was not going to school full-time, and my sister had recently been married. Even though I missed being with young people, I felt no resentment. One day, impatient for more action, I decided to drop into a travel agency and picked up a stack of brochures on Europe, Paris, in particular. After lunch while Mother did the dishes my father and I sat at the dining room table and browsed through pamphlets, planning mock excursions. It was my way of entertaining my ailing father and looking toward the future. This was my form of summer theater and my early introduction to storytelling as a caretaking skill. One weekday afternoon my parents and I were seated on the screened-in porch at our summer house. From there, on a clear day you could see out over the saltwater marshes covered with flowered water lilies to the ocean. While making "small talk" I noticed my father's feet wiggling uneasily inside his white tasseled loafers. His attention was drawn to the footstool located in the corner diagonally across the way. I meandered across the room. As I placed the footstool by his feet, he said, "I don't know how you do it, but somehow you know what I want, before I do."

Mother habitually responded well to weather. One day in April she walked with Sybil, the nurse, close by her side. "I want to try it myself instead of sitting in the rocking chair and watching you prepare the vegetables this afternoon." Sybil's hand placed gently but firmly against her back, Mother leaned against the white porcelain sink with her elbows resting on the edge, her spindlelike arms supporting her seventy-one pound body weight. Shaking slightly, her small, twisted-knuckled hands held the steel peeler as she stroked outward peeling the rough skin off a small potato. I can still see her lower lip working. Had she been holding an onion, I might not have noticed her tears.

My position at Eastland Terrace oftentimes was paving the way and then stepping back, letting my parents and the nurses take over. Like a good parent, I withdrew consciously to empower them. Fortunately, I was a born organizer. From the time I was old enough to ride the local bus alone I had my pencil case purchased for the first day of school by mid-August. Several times each school day, with sheer delight, I would organize my desktop, placing the ruler and eraser just above my number-two lead pencil, which rested squarely centered in the groove to the left of the inkwell. Every Christmas I would ask Santa for a diary with a key and a wallet, preferably red, and then that night I would snuggle up on the rose-colored couch and list my well-thought-through New Year resolutions, fill in my new identification card, and slip photographs between clear plastic slots.

As an adult I honored volunteer work as an important part of being a responsible citizen and an extension of my God-given mothering skills. Like a big mother bear I embraced positions of responsibilities at the Haverhill Girls Club. I presented organizational workshops for the Merrimack Valley United Fund. All this bolstered the skills I would need to pull the household successfully together. Now, as Mother was recuperating, I strove to create balance and harmony on a daily basis among the cast of characters in our household. If one nurse tried to tell another nurse how to run her shift, I tried to see all the way around the situation. Sitting upright in my favorite chair, I would close my eyes and rest my hands, palms up, on my lap. Breathing deeply, I would clear a peaceful space within myself. This often required patience. When I felt relaxed and focused I visualized the problem and placed it, figuratively speaking, in the center of the coffee table. Through my imagination I walked slowly and methodically around this imaginary table, examining the issue from every angle and each person's perspective. When I had finished the process, I felt confident that I had considered each individual's point of view, including my father's. This exercise had served me well when I was the first woman moderator of our church. Being a pioneer is risky business. I had feared if I did not do my job well it was possible the next time a woman moderator was suggested, she would be voted down, using my poor performance as an example. I sensed there were members of the congregation who had difficulty in accepting my status. That is why one afternoon seated in my living room I placed my own image on the coffee table and walked around my sense of myself, at the time, first from the female perspective and then from the male perspective. As problem-solving situations came up throughout my life afterward I used my imagination in a similar way. Now I applied it to help my parents. I resolved to see the nurses only in their professional roles. I decided not to become emotionally involved with their personal lives or needs. In actuality, I needed to keep this a business arrangement. It was important that my focus remain on my parents and not on socializing with the nurses. I relied on their professional training to support my resolve not even to know about their children. There was one exception. Karen was the easiest of the nurses for me to problem-solve with and touched my heart deeply. She was even-keeled, remained focused on my parents' needs, had a willingness to do her job well, and did not let control issues become a factor. The first time her daughter, eight-year-old Angela, came to visit was on an Easter Sunday. The idea of the visit was so the child could watch her mother at work. On occasion, usually during school vacations, Angela would bring my mother artwork from school and have lunch at the house with my parents. Karen and Angela adopted my parents. Later, when my father was alone, Angela came for dinner. When my mother died I sent Angela a thank-you note for "being you" and enclosed one of my Mother's lace hankies.

Throughout my life I have often asked myself the "either or" question: would I rather be liked or respected? Each day was a life-and-death situation. I tried hard to be friendly and efficient. I held the belief that the more the nurses understood my thinking process and where I placed my emphasis, the more clearly they could relate to my style of caregiving. When I took courses to better myself, I shared what I was learning in the classroom. This was my way of inviting dialogue and keeping the lines of communication not only open but also objective. Most of my classes were taken for credit toward an M.A. degree and were therapy-related. Keeping my emotions finely tuned was a top priority for me. When my mother returned from the hospital, I was in the midst of watercolor therapy. After two years of working together my instructor had expressed to me one day how in the beginning, I used to scare her half to death. She said, "You tracked every word I said, and you questioned every move I made." I knew my desire to learn was extreme, but I didn't realize I was making others uncomfortable with its intensity. That was my style with the nurses as well. My behavior was largely unconscious at the time, but as I look back I can see how with even greater passion I tracked their comments and actions to make certain that they were giving my parents sensitive as well as medical attention.

I had an uncontrollable need to do things in a detailed and complete manner and was never reluctant to work long hours to obtain the best possible results. There were times I felt I had created a monster by being so dutiful to the nurses. It was not unusual for me to get a telephone call at nine o'clock in the evening to let me know they had run out of something. I made certain it was there before 6:30 A.M. just in case my father woke at an earlier hour. Even Mother had me running like a spinning top. She preferred Vanity Fair napkins, and her grocery man did not carry them. I purchased them for her across town. Although obsessive, this was the role I wanted to play, and I knew that it was continually making a difference to them.

The nurses were a great help to my father, yet he found it difficult adjusting to a house full of women. My father was still sleeping upstairs. Each morning he came downstairs to a hearty leisurely breakfast, a treat that had only taken place previously during the summers at Rye Beach, when he had a house full of guests. My father was spending more time in his bedroom after arriving home from work. He always went directly upstairs to change into casual clothing. Mother's instincts told her he was staying up there too long, which made her think he was "up to something." My father had always been a perfect gentleman and host. This feeling of awkwardness had him taking his daily drink upstairs alone. This way he was assured more privacy and solitude. Later we surmised that it was not his intention to have "too much"; he simply couldn't remember if he had just had one, two, or more. He did not fall asleep upstairs; he came back down, as my mother feared, looking for a fight. As soon as Mother was able, she made her way to the top of the landing and into his bedroom to pour the "stuff" down the drain. From then on he had his one drink each evening in the family room, watching the evening news and reading the daily newspaper. Mother sat in her blue wingback chair next to his, tight-lipped, full of anxiety and uncertainty, waiting for "the other shoe to fall." We went through the same scenario regarding his dosages of cough syrup once when he had a sore throat and cold. During the day, employees at the dealership were finding him fast asleep at his desk in his private office. On occasion they would draw his office drapes to protect his dignity. It was a pitiful sight for me to see the grieving expressions on grown men's faces as they watched my father's unremitting deterioration.

My father was repeating himself more and more, and I had to find a way to tolerate this behavior. I discovered I could turn the situation into a game by counting on my fingers the number of ways I could answer the same question. At first I felt snippy, like a smart aleck, until I finally realized it was another of my survival techniques. My mother used a more passive form of game playing. During his tangential conversations, she would close her eyes and pretend to sleep, hoping this would discourage him from carrying on. She would sit motionless, striving to become invisible. She couldn't see him; maybe he couldn't see her? She would discourage conversation by giving one-word answers, which only agitated Father even more.

The doctor asked me to bring Mother to his office every three weeks, and I complied. Generally I was pleasant and willing to wait my turn. On one occasion I saw a former city council member walk straight in, and I lost my cool. I walked crisply to the nurses' desk and said, "If I had known all it took was a penis to be next in line, I would have brought one along." She smiled. Then, lady-like, I took my seat again. Although this comment got no immediate results, it became clear I was no pushover. During the long waits in the doctor's office, I was concerned because Mother had no bounce on her fanny. I brought in brochures from home; flipping through pages of "pretty" helped the long wait to go by faster.

One visit stands out among all the rest. Her doctor had just finished listening to her heart. My eyes were glued to his every movement. I focused on my breath.

"Things look good, Alice," he said. "I'd say you must be doing all the right things."

Her smile looked strained; she was unable to look him directly in the eyes as she buttoned her blouse."

"It's Ted," she said. "I don't know what to do. His moods can be terrible, particularly at night."

Dr. Munter fell into thought. His serious nature was what I had learned to like best about him. "You are describing Sundown Syndrome Alice. This often occurs with Alzheimer patients. I suspected Ted had Alzheimer's when you were in the hospital. The way he shuffled when he walked, his lack of memory and repetitiveness tipped me off to his condition. That's why I put up with him the way I did." I knew he was referring to my father's uncontrollable demands to make Mother better.

After the doctor had identified my father as having Alzheimer's disease, we observed his behavior with more clarity. I sensed that it was easier for Mother to know her attentive, handsome, generous, cantankerous husband could be described as having a disease rather than having to describe him as "downright hateful." Nevertheless, his behavior was increasingly an embarrassment for her in front of others. My father's personality had always been considered "feisty," particularly during the full moon. Mother never wavered in her theory that he was sometimes like his own mother. One day my grandfather George had dropped off a bag of money that my grandmother had been hoarding during her final years, at my parents' kitchen door. My father, in his need to stay on his ethical track, had my brother-in-law John count the cash, then deliver $25,000 directly to the attorney's office, to be included in her estate. That day, we *all* declared my father "downright crazy," paying money to the government when there was no need to. Sundown Syndrome is said to be related to the high percentage of water in our bodies, which is connected to the tides and the moon. I have heard nurses tell about the disturbing influences of the full moon. The stressful behavior usually occurs during late afternoon and continues throughout the night. Years back I remember the shocked response I got from Barbara when during the full moon time I said I thought Daddy was a "lunatic" because at the dealership he was changing his mind and denying what he had said only minutes previously. He would shoot nonsensical questions at me. Now I saw my father pacing the living room floor for as long as six hours at a time, continually repeating the same thought. The senseless chatter was wearing my mother down. When she attempted to distract his attention away from his thoughts, this did not make a difference to him. The following morning he had no memory of his behavior or of her efforts to calm him down. During breakfast when asked how he slept, after these ongoing repetitive bouts, he would reply, "Best night sleep I ever had."

During his periods of Sundown Syndrome, he had physical strength he did not have during the early hours of the day. It became necessary to install sliding bolted locks, out of reach, along the top moldings of the doors. The locks kept him safe by preventing him from leaving the house. Should he have managed to get out, we would have a "devil of a time" getting him back in. During my adolescent years, I remember how my father would spend his leisure time downstairs in the playroom, shooting pool, while Mother, Barbara, and I stayed upstairs in the kitchen, washing and drying the dinner dishes. He had shot pool and played cards regularly to keep his mind sharp. It broke my heart the day the cellar door was bolted and the skeleton key hidden in the wooden tray inside the kitchen dish towel drawer.

Gordon and I had seen many of our friends taking care of their older parents as they crossed the threshold; it wasn't an unusual decision when we decided to do this, too. Gordon never flinched and he never walked away during the years of my father's Alzheimer illness. My husband was my safety net. Because he was remarkably reliable I was able to persevere over such a long period of time. I knew deep down that he could finish whatever I was unable to complete. I had developed a habit over the years of really sharing my experiences with him, so it was not unusual for me to share this, too. Throughout our marriage whatever I needed to communicate to him has been patiently welcomed and tolerated with kind deep interest. He would ask daily, "How are things going at Eastland Terrace?" Most of the time I answered in detail. When it came to sharing extraordinary experiences, he maintained a steady ear. I knew it was crucial to my father's well-being and to mine that Gordon be kept up-to-date; should something happen to me he would be next "in command."

There were occasions at night when the nurses found

it necessary to call Gordon for assistance. If my father fell, it took added strength to pick him up. His body could become deadweight, yet he could be very strong. We were learning my father behaved more appropriately in the company of a man. When my father was made to feel safe, he was more apt to be good. My mother felt safer with a male family member around as well. My father's autonomy was being snatched away by strangers and a disease he had never even heard of, much less pronounced.

My father was a very challenging person even before he had Alzheimer's, yet somehow Gordon saw beyond that. I knew Gordon's role in caring for my father was difficult, but it never occurred to me that he couldn't handle it. The most he would do, even when the call came in late at night, was roll his eyes, then get dressed again and do what needed to be done. One night as I wondered if he would return home fully disheartened I read repeatedly *Omar Khayyám's* poem: "*Ah Love! could you and I with Him conspire, To grasp this Sorry Scheme of Things entire, Would not we shatter it to bits-and then, Remold it nearer to the Heart's Desire.*" When he returned home, rather than causing him to relive his experience, I simply would ask, "Is everything OK?" and he would answer, "Yes." By the miracle of his own constitution, when he'd come home after his bouts with my father's Alzheimer's, Gordon would get back in his pajamas and be asleep in five minutes. It often wasn't until a night or two later, when he volunteered to discuss his late-night visits and I saw his cheeks quiver, that I really knew how hard being there was for him, even though he did it without complaining. How hard it was to be with my father when he was being wild, when the bolts were being latched on the doors; how Gordon was being bent out of shape and what

56

a miracle it was that he was able to maintain and regain his composure.

He hid his feelings from me in his way as I hid mine, so as not to burden me with any more fears and doubts and anxieties than I already had. He knew I was already, every day, on the edge. I have grown to have a greater appreciation for his deep feelings at the time and my need for him to hide those feelings because I needed him to be steady. I can also see now how many men would not have made themselves available the same way Gordon did: they would purchase season tickets for night games or just say, "No."

My mother was from the generation that asked, "What will the neighbors think?" She was as protective of my father's community image as she was of her own. He had been diagnosed with Alzheimer's, and she was embarrassed for him. She did not want people to see how confused and unmanageable he could be. Friends, and relatives were asking when they could drop by for a visit. For Mother it was out of the question. Nevertheless, Barbara and I encouraged her to allow a short visit from her sister, who faithfully called each A.M. at 9:15 and in the late afternoons. "Just checking in," she'd say. I was surprised and pleased the day she announced that Uncle Alfred was dropping by. He was Mother's younger brother, very funny and easy to be with. Mother stood by the black chair inside the entranceway to the living room as the nurse let her brother in the back door, his eyes overflowing with tears. They hugged for a very long time. She knew he saw her as his "tough little sister." Leaning back to get a full-blown look at him, she said, "They'll have to take me out in the woods and shoot me before they'll get rid of me. I'm no sissy!"

My nephew Dana found a book on Alzheimer's and passed it around to all the family members as well as the nurses. Everyone encouraged me to read it. My instincts told me it was more important to learn storytelling skills rather than to read about Alzheimer's disease. Fearing that research data would become walls of limitation for me, I explained, "I want to visit my father as a daughter and not as a clinical technician. He has enough medical people around him now and many more available." I knew I needed to take a defensive position in order to protect my ability to generate positive energy. My attitude toward more information only increased my intention to create a full and vibrant life for us all. I became increasingly aware of the difference between clinical description and full-blown life. I did not have to look at my father to see what harmful affect Alzheimer's was having on him; all I had to do was take a look at my mother. Mother was living with the disease continuously, day in and day out. Even when she was out for a "jaunt" she couldn't help but fear what she would find at home. More and more my father was "clueless"; his lack of memory wiped out any recollection of stress. Yet, ironically, he was looking healthier by the day.

Even though Alzheimer patients share similar patterns, each individual case of Alzheimer's is unique. I preferred not to see Alzheimer's by the book but by following my own intuition. For this reason I did not attend support groups. I was also afraid I might become absorbed in the emotional states of others. Rather than diagnosing and prognosing, I turned my mind to finding supportive, creative workshops. I was in the school of life. I knew at forty-nine years of age that I was at a stage when I needed to develop some new perspective. I felt that no matter what was going on around me, I was in my own growing process and I needed to pay attention to it; otherwise, I, too, might get sick myself, and then I would be of no use to anyone. I habitually read catalogs, brochures, and inspirational books. When someone suggested a book to me I often went out and bought it. For several years I had attended educational conferences in Virginia exploring spirituality, psychotherapy, and creativity. I was especially impressed, during this difficult autumn of 1994, with Christine Northrop, creator of "Women's Bodies and Women's Wisdom" workshop, who raised the same question I, too, had been finding thought-provoking: what constitutes scientific proof? I was always driving deep for the honest answer. I was the daughter of a self-made man. I, too, was learning life on the job. Eager to teach myself to be a self-made caretaker, I was honoring that part within me to be unorthodox and authentic, like my parents. It took patience, courage, and insightful understanding to find the harmony within myself. Northrop's words helped me to feel validated. I also was strengthened by Ralph Waldo Emerson's essay "Self-Reliance."

I had learned over several years the power of positive denial, weeding out negative news. Several years previously I had established an environmental discipline, a habit of only taking in that which could benefit my growth as a human being. My father had taught me emotional discipline. If in his presence the storyline of a program had either my sister or me in tears, he would curtly say, "Turn that TV off. There is no need filling your head full of that nonsense." Now I was giving myself the same message. I watched a limited amount of TV news and only read newspaper articles that I was attracted to; this left me feeling uninformed at times compared to others.

By May 20, 1987, Mother asked to have her spring

59

clothes brought down from the attic. She was taking charge of her checkbook again, even though her eyes were failing and it took her all morning to write out a few checks. I was feeling increasingly protective and less anxious. I was examining her clothes weekly for soiled spots, as well as scrutinizing her demeanor. One day we planned a trip to have her hair permed. For fifteen years, Mother had kept a standard weekly appointment with Eleanor, who not only owned her own beauty shop but also was an accomplished oil painter and teacher, excelled in Greek cooking, and had recently graduated from Harvard University with a degree in arts and humanities. We all knew of her reputation for reading tarot cards and auras. One day, the seven-to-three regular nurse, Beth, and I were talking to Mother and Eleanor through the reflection in the large mirror in front of the salon chair where Mother was seated. Eleanor asked my mother if she wore a cross.

"No," Mother answered.

The hairdresser urged, "I wish you would. You need special protection right now." We thought of my father's irrational harassment. "It can be a very small cross, so no one can see it," she insisted. "You can just pin it to your slip strap."

Hearing this reminded me of when I was sixteen and worked at the local bank and assisted clients in opening their safe-deposit boxes. The ladies I considered the most eccentric would dig down through the necklines of their dresses in order to find the special keys they had attached to their underwear earlier.

Beth piped up, "I have plenty of crosses at home Alice. I'll bring one in tomorrow." There was a time when, in front of Mother, crosses and rosary beads made me feel uncomfortable. Mother had been excommunicated from

60

the Catholic Church when she married my Protestant father. Today was different. The reference to crosses was more a statement of spirituality and faith than that of a specific religion. As soon as I arrived home I called my children and Barbara to let them know that Eleanor had come up with an ingenious plan to protect Mother's religious inclination. Beth must have mentioned it to other nurses as well. The following morning, spread out on the blue formica kitchen counter was an assortment of crosses, all shapes and sizes, for Mother to choose from. She chose the cross that would fit most freely onto the tiniest of safety pins, which she wore until the end.

I drove Mother on her excursions. Although she maintained an erect posture, she appeared very small sitting in the front seat of my automobile. Mother never placed her pocketbook out of sight like I am apt to do, throwing mine in the backseat. She always kept her black leather bag on her lap, protected by her arthritic hands, one hand placed on top of the other. Mother had always worn stylish hats. As a child I had watched her slide her hands along the netting as she placed the veil gracefully, subtly, across her forehead or below eye level, resting on her cheekbones. Her hats were usually black or navy, although she wore a rose pillbox on the day of my sister's wedding. Mother more recently had been wearing a chenille print kerchief tied under her chin or, if it was raining, a clear plastic rain hat that was tightly pleated and when snapped would fold into a case that had the name of her local bank or insurance company stamped on it. I monitored her profile during our outings. I would make a point of noticing if her lower lip was quivering, I listened to hear if she was mumbling unintelligible words, an expression of her nervousness usually brought about by my father's erratic, unintelligible behavior the night before.

Being around my mother was like supporting a winning candidate; the stronger she became, the more committed I was to her campaign. Little by little her sense of independence returned. One day we went to the Burlington Mall, the wheelchair placed inconspicuously in the trunk. Beth, came with us in the car. We watched Mother gleefully weave in and out through the clothes racks at Lord & Taylor's. She hadn't lost her touch. In no time at all she had spotted the dress she wanted. It was navy blue knit, belted, with white pique peter pan collar and cuffs and gold buttons down the front, which meant she could step into it. With a snap of the finger she said to the clerk, "I'll take it," without even looking at the price tag. When you're considered "an exception" by your doctor, you hear your offspring telling everyone she's the daughter of "a walking miracle," you're out on a toot for the very first time in over a year, eighty-six years of age, and you know you can afford it, you see a dress you like and you want it, why not? Mother's influence was rubbing off on the nurses. Beth came back that Monday telling us about the grand old time she had shopping during the weekend. We were all learning to find the positive moment at hand. Mother was showing increasing signs of enjoyment being away from my father and out of the house. During her outings she was one of "the girls."

Fast-food joints were now at the top of her list of favorite restaurants. I enjoyed seeing her eating enthusiastically, even a less than healthy burger smothered with ketchup, and accompanied with french fries. Halfway through lunch, she would hand me a ten-dollar bill. Mother realized she was out of touch with prices. She would give me more than enough money. As she placed the folded money in my hand, she would invariably say, "Don't forget your father's apple turnover. He'll be looking for a present just like he did in the old days." This was a reference to her shopping trips to Boston. Anything she bought she had sent home, for the sake of convenience and confidentiality, with the exception of a new necktie for my father. With childlike anticipation he'd ask, "Did you buy me a tie?" She'd respond, giving him her usual answer, "It's on the table next to your chair." Only at Christmastime would she alter this routine, with: "You'll have to wait for Santa." He'd reply with, "Well, he better hurry up. I'm running short."

On August 29, 1988, my father had prostate surgery. The "girls" were now focusing more of their nursing skills on my father than my mother. His diagnosis was now familiar to us all, yet after his prostate operation he stayed home for good. The daytime nurses who attended to my mother were not used to caring for him at home because he usually had been at the car dealership. When he came home from the hospital the nurses had to start putting incontinence garments on him. Before, he had always gone upstairs himself to change into comfortable clothes; the first six months he stayed away from work, he continued to dress in a sport coat and tie. His style of attire charmed everyone. My father insisted, as of yet, he had not decided whether or not to retire. He said he was staying home "checking out" how well the business could run without him. I imagined their mixed emotions when the salesmen and customers at the dealership got wind of his stepping down. My father had been actively there for sixty-eight years; his absence would signify the end of an era. Yet my father's unpredictable Alzheimer behavior had been reaching its boiling point for quite some time.

He had been causing embarrassing moments and major interruptions. People were kind and understanding, but clearly much of his behavior now was definitely unsuitable to a business environment. Our daughter Valerie tells about a time when she was home on college break and was working at the dealership. She recalls with a smile, "I never was fortunate enough to get a job answering the phone or working in the sales room. I was cleaning my uncle's office. He had asked if I would please wash his ficus plant. I got a glimpse of Grandpa looking at me from across the showroom, and the next thing I knew he was headed in my direction yelling and cursing at me and saying 'Is this what I pay you for around here? You get out of here; you just get out of here. You're not worth anything around here. Furthermore, you're fired!' " Valerie understood he didn't mean all that he was saying. "I could tell by the hazy look in his eyes he no longer knew who I was or what I was doing there. My previous experience with Grampa had also told me it was possible he might not have known where he was himself, even though he had been able to navigate about his building. I felt devastated and humiliated to think that my grandfather had just fired me in front of all his employees and customers. What was Grammie going to think? I did not want my experience to upset her. To think only a few hours ago Grampa and I had been talking about school life and my selected courses. He always took great interest in what I was learning. The next day when I went to drop something off at my grandmother's house, I said I was no longer working down at the garage. She responded by saying, 'Yes, I know, but that's OK.' I could tell by the resigned tone in her voice that she had not wanted to talk about it any longer. Over the years my grandmother had made a habit of 'sticking up' for my grandfather, even when she didn't agree with him. It was a silent code and I respected her kind of loyalty."

Years back Mother had kept in touch through a morning talk show host, a family psychologist. She observed trends and listened without judgment, which allowed her mind to accept new ideas. Now on days we were alone I'd asked, "Is there something you would like to get off your chest today?" One morning, after an evening when Gordon had spent several hours helping to calm my father, I asked Mother if she would like to see a therapist: "Sometimes we need people other than family to talk to, and I want you to have an opportunity to let it all out. You seldom cry and maybe you should."

Her tone was calm but sad: "I am too old to air my linens, and I could never talk badly about your father to a stranger."

My father always said, "You cannot expect sick people to make decisions for themselves." His words were the only permission I needed. I set about visiting nursing homes, placing his name on the waiting lists of those I thought the rest of the family would approve. I waited for the right moment to tell my mother what I was doing. One morning, after she had had another difficult evening with my father and Sundown Syndrome and asked for Gordon's help and he returned home and gave a play-by-play description of what had gone on, I realized it had reached its boiling point. The following morning I said, "Mother, I understand your reasoning in not wanting to see a therapist. Freedom of choice is very important for me, too."

Her facial expression had changed over the past three years. When I mentioned the word *choice,* I saw the deep, enduring lines on her face filling in with a smoother, gentler softness.

"Mother," I said, "I have Daddy on the waiting list in

five nursing homes. All you have to do is give us the word, and the family will take care of the rest." She never did.

Actions are like ideas thrown to the wind; my visits were now designed to fill my parents' days with joy, companionship, memories, and laughter. My father would be seated in his regular chair at the kitchen table and Mother, as usual, next to him. Because I had a good memory, an eye for detail, and the gift of gab, I was able to use family albums effectively as a resource for storytelling. Each snapshot was a story in itself, which I exploited to its fullest possibility. I chose less recent albums, where my parents, and their friends looked healthy, poised, and cavalier. Mother and I would speak of the old hats and positive pleasant moments. My husband's family had a collection of old postcards he found in our attic. These also came in handy. On rare and special days, our laughter started deep and grew into hilarity that caused our eyes to water.

I was a continuing education student in Cambridge, Massachusetts. Many of my class exercises seemed extreme to suburban folk. One morning I announced I was going to show them what I had learned in Storytelling through Movement class the night before. The nurse looked around for the best vantage point. I was going to need room, lots of it. I moved Mother's rocker into the dining room. All eyes were on me. At that moment I liked my show better than conversation. With a full inhalation I stretched my body toward the ceiling; then I quickly rolled it downward. "The wave begins to open, you can see the white foam along the top," I shouted, and with bended knees I threw my outstretched arms upward and swished across the kitchen floor, roaring, a monstrous act of nature fighting to survive in a deadly storm.

My father's response was predictable. He roared out loud, "Wonderful!"

Mother with a crooked smile simply said, "Jesus, Mary, and Joseph, there she goes again."

My life had become like "Little Black Sambo," a favorite childhood tale of mine, in which the tigers ran round and round until they melted into a pool of butter. I was running around-the-clock, meeting each parent's individual needs. Yet the situation was too grave for me to let myself go any further off balance. On days when I was moving especially quickly, I would look to see if I was in harmony with my surroundings. When circumstances fell into place naturally, I took that as a good sign. Years previously, when I had studied Carl Jung and his dream works. I had come across his "synchronicity" theory, linking inner and outer events. I knew it was going to be a good day when my misplaced half-slip appeared shiny on top of a pile stacked high with unfolded laundry. With my eyes rolled upward and a playful grin on my face, I said out loud, "Thank You, Lord."

Sometimes in those days I was a dynamo of will and determination. I found myself in the grip of spiritual forces, praying all the time for my parents and for my own inner strength. There were days in the middle of winter so filled was I with the heat and spirit of my role that I felt no need for a coat. I would bring it with me, but instead of putting it on I would fling it on the seat beside me. Mother would scold, "Where is your coat? You're going to catch your death of cold." Yet I knew differently, wrapped so tightly in duty and the inspiration of the moment.

As my mind awakened each morning, I heard myself whisper in silence, *This is the day the Lord has made; rejoice and be glad in it.* Immediately I put on my rose-colored glasses. I realize now that I was exercising my power to make my life work through positive denial. I kept my glasses firmly in place when I went into town to shop or to a local restaurant. On my worst days, if they slipped, old friends and acquaintances appeared uglier than anything that was happening in our household. How painful it was for me to see their pity for "the poor Marble family." A spark of anger would flare in my head when they questioned, "does your father remember your name?" Although my parents were nearing ninety years of age, many people acted as though death knocking at our door was a great surprise. They knew my parents were people of principle, discipline, and intelligence. Could they not see we were determined to live life fully in the shadow of death? Instead it seemed to me they wanted to insult my genuine joy at serving my parents. I put my glasses back on and attempted to ignore them.

There were days when I found it extremely painful to drive up my parent's street to see people from the area walking their dogs, who knew perfectly well what was happening but never took the time to wave me down and speak with me. Oftentimes my disappointment turned into a headache. I'd slow my car and volunteer a report to lighten my fury. My visits to my parents usually took place at the kitchen table, by a large picture window. From that vantage point we could see the neighborhood. Many times my parents smiled and prepared to wave, only to find people who could see my parents clearly in the kitchen window, ignore them. I wanted to open the window and scream, "Are you blind?" How painful and sad it was for me to see my courageous parents yearning to feel part of the neighborhood, if only in a small way. I often held back my tears. As my parents' illness dragged on, the neighbors ignored us more and more thoroughly. One lady sat silently on her front porch as I entered the house shortly after my mother died, as if I did not exist. I know now these people were wearing their own tinted glasses and clouding us out. I did not want to be vengeful; instead I would make little bargains with myself. I bought food treats, clothing treats as well.

Gordon fathered my parents with protectiveness and muscular strength. Mothering them was grinding me down. I would feel pain in my hands from giving. Seeing that I needed to treat myself with the same respect I used as I cared for others, I began to give my aching hands special attention. For years I had avoided wearing perfume. The only time I wore it was when I did heavy housecleaning and it made me feel more like the "lady of the house." I bought scented hand cream and massaged my hands while watching evening television. During the day I dialogued with my hands. I would tell them how grateful I was for their sturdiness, even though I could feel them tied up in knots. I thanked them on a spiritual level as well for hours at my parents' kitchen table, dancing around my words, eloquently expressing my love. One day, when my left hand was hurting badly, I asked, "Is there anything I can do for you?" *Yes,* it replied. *Slow down.*

In those days, I wasn't able to slow down in the way I have learned to today. So I took a pair of skin-tight kid gloves, ones I had worn to weddings years before, and cut the fingertips off at the top. This way I was able to do my household chores. As bizarre as this sounds, it gave me the message to treat my hands more gently, which in turn eased the pain. I trained myself not to feel ashamed of taking care of the caretaker any more than I was ashamed of caring for my parents.

For years under pressure my pattern had been to develop a headache, which lasted as long as twenty one days. During these six years these migraines persisted. When I look back I can see that my headaches obstructed some of my feelings, especially my sorrow and anger. Anger is like an afflicted heart. I would boil up and get head pressure by not dealing with the anger. The seed of sorrow is in the lungs. The sadness was pressing in my chest cavity and pushing it up. This was the easiest way for my energy to move. I was steaming mad a lot of the time, but I was not conscious of that. On some days I would take as many as three baths. I could see what the water was doing for me in these fiery circumstances. My bathing routine was like going into the bathroom and locking the door as mothers do when they don't get any peace from their children. To my warm bath I would add cupfuls of fragrant oils, scents that were warm, grounding, and soothing, like sandalwood, Jojoba bath gel and rose geranium. Today I am attracted to the lighter side of life; I choose sweeter scents, like, lily of the valley and Persia lilac. These long and leisurely baths would bring me down into my breathing and inner circulation.

Someone had to be in charge. I learned to relax out of my routine walks. I went places where I wouldn't be found. If I thought my family expected me to be walking in one direction, I took another. I was distancing myself. There were times the lump that sat in my throat was too big to swallow. I couldn't digest, one more time, hearing the phone ring. I was as anxious to be asked to pick up a quart of milk, as I was to hear that I had lost one of my parents.

Winter or summer, three or four times a week, I took the thirty-five-minute drive to the beach to walk along the sand when only runners and nighttime fishermen would be present. Standing still at the shoreline, my eyes closed, I inhaled slowly and deeply, making each moment last. I could feel the essence of salt water, healing every cell of my weary body.

One day I noticed that when other members of the family came for visits they received the same gratifying response from my parents as I did. Yet they were doing little to maintain the household as they breezed in and out, from my perspective, choosing the path of least resistance. I began to notice how they positioned themselves differently in a chair. An active person sits more near the edge of his seat, shoulders leaning back but upright, in a state of readiness. The less driving person sits with his lower spine tucked into the crevice where the seat and back of the chair meet, shoulders resting. I felt envious and somewhat resentful. I did not want to harbor any anger. I also did not want to have this turn me bitter and grumpy. I would need a preventative plan. That is when I got the idea to pay myself twenty-five dollars a week from my joint checking account with Gordon. Two years later, when Mother and I were upstairs in the sitting room chatting, by accident I let my salary arrangement slip out. We were together a lot in those days and I was always looking for something to talk to her about.

"You what?" she said with raised eyebrow. "From now on take it out of the grocery money."

My father was a man who had lived by rules of law and order. Now he was throwing off the family's equilibrium. One day I wanted to be able to give my mother more realistic support and to give those who asked questions a more descriptive and satisfying answer. My storytelling background told me it could be helpful to think in metaphors. It was then I remembered being told by the doctor to imagine the Alzheimer patient's mind as a whole pie sliced into eight separate pieces, each piece disassociated from the other. Staying focused on that analogy, I realized that my father's mind did not have all the connecting pieces and that no one, including my father, could successfully predict which piece would function.

I persevered until I came up with three guidelines to hold onto. I wrote these out:

1. Accept the situation however illogical it is.
   I wanted to deny the illness in order to create normalcy, yet there was my father seated in his own living room, feeling angry and wanting to go home.
2. Remember the disease allows Daddy to do only one thing at a time.
   The house was a catalyst for a lot of activity. I was aware my father had difficulty in following a three-way conversation. For that reason, I left when others stopped by. When my father was still active and running in and out of the house doing errands, Mother left his car keys on the corner of the dining room table along with some mail that was to be taken to the dealership. Her taking care of him in this way had become a regular practice. I heard her say, "Ted, don't forget to pick up the fish at Herb's Market before you come home." His response was the usual, "I will." Mother continued, "By the way, also speak to Eleanor about sending home my allowance." Eleanor was the car dealership's bookkeeper, who had administered my father's checkbook for years. I could clearly hear the frustration in his voice when he answered, "Wait a minute; wait a minute, Al. I can only do one thing at a time. You call Eleanor yourself."
3. Daddy's world has no space or time. Stay with the moment.
   For years I had tried many forms of meditation, including fishing. Now my father was conveying to me his final teaching. Live life in the moment! I saw him increasingly as universal life and less as a man with a

disease. Sitting across from my father sometimes became a cosmic experience. My limited studies in Zen had taught me, "We are life and life is limitless." I would focus on an invisible beam connecting our thoughts, never letting my eyes leave his as he, too, stared into my eyes, working hard to communicate.

I knew my father's life had been permanently changed when I saw him using white Kleenex to wipe his nose rather than his traditional white hand-rolled, initialed handkerchief. Now he was wearing his Kleenex in his shirt breast pocket. In the past when he was going off to work each day he carried his hanky in his back trouser pocket. Like both my parents, I was an extremely observant child. As a youth, I remember first thing in the morning when I would have been headed for the bathroom, passing by my parents' bedroom door I would see my father all dressed up with suit and tie, standing in front of his bureau dabbing a few drops of cologne on his handkerchief before placing it, nicely folded, in his back pant pocket. The cologne was in a square bottle with a gold dome screw top and a brown jockey hat and crop on the front of the label. His next ritual would be to place the loose change on his bureau in his left-side pant pocket. He would stand there for a split second determining if the coins were too heavy. I hoped they were because then I knew he would give Barbara and me the excess. His car keys he popped underneath the flap of his jacket and into his pocket.

My father changed when he wasn't a businessman needing to stay on top of company matters. My sister and John bought him a free-standing bird feeder, which they positioned outdoors, in the side yard, diagonally across from where he sat at the kitchen table. He delighted in the humor of the squirrels and the wisdom of the birds. He was intent on details. His capacity for exact observation of people, places, things, voices, and attitudes was a practiced skill. Sometimes he was able to peel back his armor and allow his sense of humor to surface. There was always a lesson to his humor, which was open and allowed dialogue. He wasn't trying to merely amuse us. My mother had never been with him at home all day before, and he broke her routine. She was eighty-eight and not flexible. Aware of how fragile and run-down her nervous system had become, she would do anything to avoid confrontation. In the middle of the kitchen, my father would say playfully, with his usual warm, winning smile, "You're looking good, Al." She would reply with a tilt of her hand, an uncertain smile, "Oh, hush up, Ted." Her temperament became increasingly introverted. Holding his uncertainty and her fear, Mother lost the ability to exhale freely and to relax. She could never tell how long his sense of humor would last or at what point it could reverse itself and become an attack on her. His wit felt unsafe. Mother oftentimes used avoidance as a way of managing her own vulnerability. She didn't look him straight in the eye anymore but cast her glance off to his right side, unless her anger and frustration reached its boiling point. Then she gave him the same glaring stare she had given me when I was a child, dining in public, and had forgotten to place my napkin in my lap.

Gordon for years referred to my car as "Janet's office": library books strewn across the passenger side of the station wagon, peach pits, lollypop sticks, and chewing gum wads filling the ashtray, panty hose rolled up and tucked under the driver's seat. Now my mother was using my car as her headquarters for talking over family business. Having the nurses under foot, twenty-four hours a day, for close to two years, my mother was missing privacy in her home.

After my father's prostate surgery, Mother slept upstairs and my father took over her bed downstairs in the family room. As she reclaimed her health and authority, she turned to business matters of the household. Firm and focused, she geared up to take charge, very organized and proud of her management skills. "You do what you have to do" was her philosophy. When Barbara and I were younger, my mother was the one who chased the yellow jackets with the fly swatter while my father sat reading his paper, watching his wife in amusement. She set the mousetraps down in the cellar and telephoned the exterminator when one was required. She enjoyed her interaction with household businesspeople and was very likeable, and people enjoyed working for her. She always paid her bills on time, and they knew that.

During the autumn of 1988 Mother sensed that she was going to die, and "doing business" was all part of her preparation. The date and time of my mother's death were not important to her, but having her house in order was. One Thursday the New England fall foliage was too picturesque to take Mother directly home from the hairdresser's. Instead we headed ten miles out of town to Barker's roadside stand for some fresh vegetables. I was surprised to hear her say, "I have put our Florida apartment up for sale. Tomorrow a realtor will put a price on the furnishings and the rest of the contents." Then my mind flashed on the asparagus dish I had bought for my father one Christmas. I could see vividly the two-section dish sitting upright in the china cabinet inside the condo. My father had always loved Arthur Godfrey, a popular radio entertainer of his generation who had his audience howl about soggy tea bags while he sold tea very effectively. That Christmas I bought my father a small silver tea bag strainer with matching saucer. The following year I bought the French hand-painted dish for asparagus, which allowed the excess juices to drain. I pulled the car over to a scenic place in the road where we could talk "business" and have the benefit of eye contact.

"I'm impressed; you have found the stamina to deal with other matters as well as Daddy," I said, anxious to give my mother words of empowerment.

"That's not all," she continued. "I have spoken to Eleanor at the garage, and she has lined up the attorney to come to the house someday next week. There are two items I want to change in our will. Because your father can only manage one thing at a time, I will have to have the lawyer come back a second time. Every night I go over the changes with your father. So far, he is going along with me."

My father had oftentimes praised my mother in public for the way she managed the household. Now in their last days together my father was relying on his wife's good sense to do what was right for them.

I, too, hoped to do what was right by not asking my mother for details. Later I learned the codicil to the will had been to increase the amount of money to be left to their seven loving and faithful grandchildren. Mother died before the second change could be executed. As her life forces waned, the grandchildren bolstered her. There was a pleasure in that exchange. She would hear their entertaining tales with a soft nonjudgmental ear. Her open-mindedness was what kept the children coming back. It was early in November when my mother telephoned her three granddaughters and set a special date and time to have them meet at her house. The children were used to dropping in one at a time, but never before had their grandmother asked them to come as a group. I heard later that when they arrived at the house my mother directed them upstairs to her bedroom, where she had spread out along the foot of her twin bed her life-long accumulation of jewelry. I can imagine the scene: the girls full of giggles, nudging one another as they tried to get a peek at themselves in the long mahogany mirror above the bureau. What fun it must have been to see how they looked in the same jewelry they had seen so often on their grandmother. I am sure my mother was brimming with pleasure that afternoon, seeing her treasured pins, necklaces, and earrings giving such pleasure to her three little women. My daughters and their cousin Melinda left the house, that autumn day, with a weighty brown paper lunch bag.

It was not unusual to have my mother ask me to go with her to the attic. Since she had taken ill she felt uneasy up there alone. She was too private a person to ask one of the nurses; it was the only area in her house that had not been handed over to them. Going to the third floor was like climbing a staircase to a sort of heaven; we could talk privately without having to keep our voices low.

This was her attic and she was in charge. I still smile when I remember her demeanor that day. She headed to Doja's room, where she had been storing her off-season clothes in jumbo garment bags. Immediately she sat down on the edge of the maple bed. Behind her were piles of freshly starched and pressed doilies and bureau scarves, the "just in case the others get soiled or turn gray" batch. As she sat, her cane hugging her side, her hand was positioned on the handle in such a way that I could see she was on a mission. "Janet," she said, "I want you to open the wicker sewing basket standing over there against the wall and empty its contents. You will find it has a fake bottom that I once put there myself. Bring to me the two envelopes you'll find in there. If I remember correctly, one is filled with canceled bank books and the other is filled with money."

My first thought was, *What will my father say if he suddenly recovers and walks in on us?* I recalled the time, just prior to Christmas, when my mother walked in unexpectedly and found my friend Jane and me sitting on the floor with all my gifts unwrapped and the boxes opened. The moment Jane saw her, she jumped to her feet and ran right past her, down the stairs, out the door, and all the way home.

I admired the way Mother turned her back on me while she counted the money and thumbed through her savings books. She was a person who did not like to be rushed, even back when she was young, wiry, and shy. This explained, in part, her need to think ahead and be organized. I was inclined to make nervous chatter, but her intense concentration told me it would be best for her if I remained quiet. It felt like an hour, but it was probably more like ten minutes before the silence was broken.

She spoke first: "Janet, what I have here is my tuck-away money of several years. It's not much." She paused. "For years you have heard me say, 'Share and share alike,' but today I want you to take a portion of this." After a pause she quickly added, "There is no need for you to mention this to your father." I removed the cold cash from her hand with the same reverence I might lift the cubed bread from a communion tray. Saying, "Thank you," didn't feel right. I simply slipped the money into my skirt pocket. Ordinarily she would have suggested, "It's time you get home to your family," but today was an exception;

neither one of us was anxious to leave this cozy space and return to the world below.

My mother never spoke about the people she admired as her role models. She was more her own person. I wanted to emulate her. From a family of nine, weaker and smaller than the others, she, as the petite one of the family, had developed a special kind of resilience and independence. She had a drive to make her own life. My father the self-made man and my mother the resilient runt: I can see how that combination was a powerful model for me in my own life. Back in the days when Calvin Coolidge was president, my mother asked to have her own money, above and beyond her weekly allowance, from my father. Money to do with what she wanted with no questions asked. The amount of money was incidental; ten cents was fine with her. I smile at the irony: ten cents was also what they paid for the bus fare the day they rode off to Salem to get married. My father loved to boast about how his feisty Irish wife recorded each weekly payment from him in her black-and-white-checked composition notebook, the same soft-bound notebook most of us carried in grade school. Because this story brought a smile to both of my parents' faces, each in different ways, it was a family tale often told around their kitchen table, before and after Mother's death.

Mother had everyone asking, "How does she do it? How does she keep herself positive?" I heard her tell a friend one day, "I won't allow myself to get down. With the situation being so bad, I am afraid I would not be able to pull myself back up."

On November 8, 1988, I flew out of Logan Airport, headed down south to my parents' Florida condominium. I especially wanted to pick up the asparagus dish and other keepsakes. The manager of the complex ushered me to my parents' unit. I was startled to see how much the condo had slipped in the eight years since I had been there. My parents were people who had kept their homes up and in good repair. They were from the old days, when cleanliness was next to godliness. Now their condominium looked dreary. It lacked the clean crispness my mother's home once had. The upholstery not only was badly faded but also had several stains. When the manager asked if I would like to have the metal shutters removed from the porch and window areas to let more light in, I graciously said, "No thank you." The artificial light was showing me even more than I cared to see. I was in the kitchen area, stirring a glass of iced tea, when I realized my parents had been failing for more years than I thought. Mother's diminishing eyesight had taken its toll. The kitchen area was not clean by my mother's standards. The paper had not been changed in the kitchen drawers for a very long time. The countertops felt unsanitary. The teapot on the stove lacked luster. A feeling of sadness overwhelmed me. I called Gordon and told him I would be home sooner than I had expected. I slept, both nights, on the living room couch.

To shake things up and get them moving a bit after the holidays that year, I came up with the idea of having a "bash" to celebrate my parents' anniversary. The only problem was it was their sixty-ninth anniversary, which was a rather odd number for the gala affair that I was envisioning. I told their friends it was their seventieth anniversary in order to get their full attention. We placed the announcement in our church newsletter, knowing our faithful, supportive church family would pull together by sending cards and congratulatory messages. At the garage, Eleanor, the bookkeeper, posted an announcement

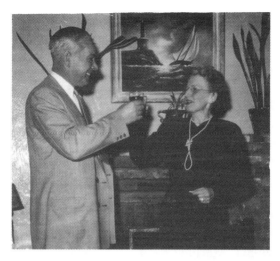

My parents toasting with cola on their anniversary

and their home address next to the time clock. I knew we could count on loyal friends to get the word out as well. On the great day, the nurses decorated the kitchen with crepe paper streamers, balloons, and a HAPPY ANNIVERSARY sign, which hung along the picture window next to the breakfast table. I asked the luncheon be catered by Irma Hale, a friend of my parents who had celebrated many occasions with them, including their grandchildren's weddings. Irma kindly came early. My father accepted her kisses as warmly as Mother did. All the children, grandchildren, spouses, and nurses began to arrive by 11:30. The only people missing were our son, Jeff, who was at work in England, and Barbara's son Duncan, who was at school taking exams. The dining room kept open serving until one o'clock, to support everybody's lunch hour and also to have everything over and cleaned up before my father's Sundown Syndrome kicked in. My father enjoyed an opportunity to eat. This was the perfect timetable for him.

The next morning, anxious to review the events of the day before, I arrived at Eastland Terrace even earlier than usual. My father was dozing in his chair in the living room, so Mother and I stationed ourselves at the kitchen table as we so often did.

I said, "Mother, wasn't yesterday fun?"

"Yes, but . . ."

"But what?" I asked.

"I didn't want to tell you before now, because you were having too much fun, but it was not our seventieth anniversary, Janet."

"It wasn't, Mother?"

"No, your father and I have been married only sixty-nine years."

"Oh, no!" I exclaimed. "Oh well, in reality what difference does it make? All it means is that we celebrated it a year early."

"That's not true," she said.

"What do you mean, Mother?"

"It matters a lot, because what you did is make me a year older!"

We relaxed our weekday schedule on weekends. Elizabeth faithfully arrived Saturday mornings at seven and stayed until Sundays at three. A former nun, she had worn the black robes of the Bon Secours sisters for thirty-six years. Now she worked as a director of patient and family services at a rehabilitation hospital. My father and Elizabeth had a special rapport from the very beginning. When my father was no longer able to recall names and the days of the week, on many a day he would ask my mother, "Is the old-timer coming today?"

I still smile when I remember Elizabeth telling my father one morning how she came to leave the sisterhood. My father, a businessman that he was, asked, "How much money did they give you when you left?"

She replied, "Not a nickel."

Needless to say, my father's eyes opened wide in astonishment. "What will you do for money?" he asked.

"God will provide," she answered.

"He should," was my father's reply. "All those years you worked for Him for nothing."

On Saturdays my father liked to dress in his sporty attire: pastel slacks, loafers, a yellow buttoned boucle golf sweater. His step lightened. During the afternoons professional golf tournaments on TV invigorated him. He took delight in watching "pool sharks" like Willie Masconi and Minnesota Fats. Elizabeth and Mother would sit at the kitchen table and talk. I was grateful she could sometimes share with Elizabeth what she couldn't share with us. While Mother coddled her weekly cocktail of whiskey and ginger ale, my father was unable to tolerate any alcohol, but Elizabeth found her own method of getting around that. She would take a standard-size cocktail glass, put butter around the edge so it would hold sugar, freeze it, and then put the whiskey on the rim of the glass so that my father could taste it. When he said to Elizabeth, "This tastes weak," she would answer him by saying, "Well, I can smell it. Can't you smell it, Ted?" He never had a complaint about the popcorn. Mother was still serving her traditional Saturday night dinner of hot dogs and beans. Father was asking, "Is there plenty of ketchup in the house?" During the evening hours Elizabeth and my parents watched their weekly quota of TV, sitting in the family room, howling over the humor and antics of the current popular TV show, *The Golden Girls.*

For years my family had designated Sunday as "Family Day." Usually I stayed at home with Gordon and our children. I could count on a reliable routine continuing at my parents' house. The Sunday papers were delivered by a paperboy; the scent of crisp bacon permeated the air. Although Monday through Friday the household went by the standard rules of low cholesterol and proper diet, on Sunday mornings Elizabeth would serve eggs and bacon. After breakfast things were cleared away, and the three of them would sit at the table together. Elizabeth, the newspaper spread out in front of her, would read aloud to my father. Although he could see his watch, his eye–mind coordination made it impossible for him to read a series of words. Elizabeth was a storyteller in her own right. She held my father's interests by taking current political issues and relating them to past events. She would talk about the days of Franklin Roosevelt or the simpler times during the days of the Great Depression. Mother sat close by reading the daily papers with her magnifying glass.

During the afternoons, Elizabeth took them for rides in the car as often as she could. As Mother became more active, Elizabeth took them to restaurants as well as her house. When Mother dressed to go out, everything had to be just so. She wore her watch, her rings, and a broach. Strangers said how much she looked like Rose Kennedy, mother of the president. Eating out could be a catch twenty-two situation for Mother. It was nice to be out among a crowd of people, but my father's unpredictable behavior made her nervous and caused her to lose her appetite. When the three of them were in a restaurant and Mother and Elizabeth started to talk, he would say angrily, "Is this a private conversation?" His sarcastic manner oftentimes extended to the waitress and hostess and humiliated Mother.

Even though I worked hard not to have a personal relationship with the nurses, their stories would trickle in and sometimes erupt into ours. I don't know what happened in Beth's heart and mind. What began as a positive relationship turned into a dark battle. Perhaps she was jealous of Elizabeth's camaraderie. Perhaps Beth was stressed in her personal life. One of our few nurses who wasn't an R.N., she had decided to go for her nursing degree. She rushed my parents in order to have study time. Her son was getting ready to go to college. I was shocked when she insisted he telephone home every few hours from his senior prom although she said he was "a good boy." One day I walked into the house and saw my mother sitting in the den with a TV table pushed tightly in front of her chair. Beth was forcing her to eat cold beef stew against her will. My mother was already being bullied by my father, and I didn't want Beth adding to her stress. He had such difficulty adjusting to change, it made Mother hesitant to replace Beth. The situation was increasingly upsetting to me. My mother didn't miss a thing, yet I could see how she chose not to cause any trouble. In this three-way power struggle I stepped back. The situation took its toll on me and everybody. My anxiety pushed me into being extremely vigilant. I started to call the house punctually asking questions. I chose my words carefully: "Did Mother have an appetite this morning?" At first I had made an effort to empower Beth. When fire meets fire you have fireworks. As our wills became more locked, there were times I had an impulse to punch her hard enough to send her clear across the kitchen floor. She tried to win the afternoon nurses to her side, but they wouldn't play the game. I was reluctant to "fire" her, because I wanted my mother to be in charge. It took time for Mother to see how Beth's behavior was draining the whole household.

What do you do when you have a major personality conflict on your hands? My father's principle was altruistic: when someone was not working to his standards, he assumed there might be some way he was responsible for the situation that he did not yet understand. My mother followed his principle in relationship to Beth. I was immensely relieved when Mother finally recognized that it was time to ask Beth to leave her employment. To push matters along, one fair day in spring I said, "I will bring a large piece of paper with a line drawn down the middle and we will write down Beth's good points and other points." At nursing services we gave what we hoped a balanced picture to her supervisors of the "primary care" nurse who had been with us for a year and a half. My father's moral principal sounded within me: "I hope you will have Beth placed elsewhere within the week." I didn't want to be all responsible for her being out of work for long. I sensed she was overtired, and besides, I realized she had been with us too long. Some months later, when Mother died, Beth and I embraced and cried.

When I was exasperated and disappointed with my parents and sometimes at my wits' end, I always controlled my emotions. This, however, took a toll on me. As stressful situations built up, emotions, especially anger, began to surface in an unaccustomed way. A person with a strong, fiery sense of purpose, I am not easily distracted. I carry through to the end. As I cared for my parents from day to day I lived a very strong principle. "I will act in such a way that I will not have any regrets." One day I began to notice that I was bruising from bumping into doorjambs and hurting my hand as I turned off the water faucet. I yanked myself with a strap to my pocketbook on the back door knob. I found grease on my long skirts from not tucking before closing the car door. One week I lost my wallet twice. It was hard for me to interpret what was happening because I was living at such a high pitch. I was spinning so fast, day after day, that my orbit was beginning to wobble. One morning I sat down to take stock of my behavior. Until then, each morning upon rising I would remain in bed, with two pillows supporting my back, my legs folded in a Buddha position, and meditate for several minutes. This practice I had maintained over several years. And now, by some unknown process, I realized it had slipped away.

For many years I had worked to master my fears and other strong emotions. I had trained myself to overcome many fears. Since childhood I had feared cats. In my midforties, when a family with six cats moved in next door, I had difficulty going in and out of my own house. I knew I had to face my fear. One weekend I visited Gordon's sister, who had a cat and three daughters. The girls were only of grammar school age, yet they respected my fear. I had introduced my nieces to petting zoos and butterflies painted on their baby fingers. It only seemed natural that they should introduce me to their love of cats. Just before dinner I announced, "Tonight is the night I'm going to pat a cat." We put together a plan. When I mustered enough courage, I was to call out, "Now." It was then they would place the cat on my lap. I remember the aquamarine upholstered chair, the fluffy white cat, the girls on bended knees, huddled close by my side. I had my three fingers lined up in a row, ready to stroke Chantel's back, when I lost my nerve. The girls had to carry their pet away. So I took myself in hand. I went to the children's section of the library rather than the adult section. Even though the illustrations made my stomach turn, the reality of the drawings made my understanding of cats more vivid. I had not realized there were so many kinds of cats. While flipping through the pages I found a reasonably attractive cat. She was a soft shade of brown, cinnamon, with a full face, pale red mouth, and long eyelashes. I checked the book out with the librarian and brought her home. My problem was, where to put her? I decided to place her on the front hall table, where I could observe her during my coming and going. I pressed the pages firmly open, leaving them flat and accessible to pat. By repeatedly confronting my fear, I was able to disarm it. The process took ten days. Later when I found myself face-to-face with a cat in my yard, I talked my way to my car, saying, "I wonder what kind of a cat you are, and if you are somewhere in my book?"

Uncontrollable fear also nearly conquered me when I was thirty-five and took up skiing to be active with my husband and three children. There is one universal rule for anyone who skis: you are responsible for yourself and your equipment. I thought this was an appropriate way to teach children independence. It was not unusual to see at the base of the mountain a three- or four-year-old dragging his skis along and carrying his boots, if only by a shoelace. One day I made a realistic assessment of my attitude toward skiing. Skiing was great, as long as my two feet were on the ground. The chair lifts terrified me. Regardless of the number of times I took the chair, I would call out, "First time rider." I hoped this would cause the attendant to slow down the chair. My cordiality worked on days when business was slow. I preferred to ride the chair alone, rather than to sit next to someone who might either talk, scratch, or sneeze, causing the chair to sway. I always sat in the center of the chair. I rode the lift with my eyes closed, knees pressed properly together, arms outstretched, in opposite directions, holding tightly onto each armrail, my skis dangling down below, somewhere in outer space. I didn't want to look up; it was too high. I didn't want to look down; it was too steep. If someone called out my name or announced he was going in for lunch, I didn't answer. I simply sat frozen. It is no wonder I never saw the other skiers pulling down the overhead bar.

Gradually my fear of heights escalated and my tears poured forth more frequently. My blood rose and flooded my whole head. I developed headaches. I could go from a calm, natural state of 1 to an intensity of 10 in the flash of a second. The sensation started low in my belly and steamed me up. I decided to take private ski lessons on Saturday mornings. The first day I met John, my instructor, a fatherly figure, I said, "What I need is someone to guide me up the chair and help me to rise above my fear." John had a head cold that day. I thought he was reaching for his hanky. Instead he pulled down a sturdy, heavy bar! In a soft and kindly voice he told me to relax my shoulders and rest my feet on the lower extended bar. It was during our brown bag lunch, in the lodge, I discovered Gordon had been familiar with the overhead bar all along. Because he never used it, he never bothered informing me about it. One weekend in 1973, the same weekend Lyndon Johnson died, I stayed home from the ski slopes reading newspaper articles, watching Lady Bird and her two girls on television. Rather than continue to be at the mercy of my fear, I decided to do what I liked best. That night I approached the dinner table full of vim and vinegar, ready to give lessons on history in the making. It was only a short while later when I noticed the bored expressions, the automatic up-and-down nodding of their heads. The family had no interest in listening to what I had to say. They were too wrapped up in moguls, trails, and ski conditions. I was being left out, and understandably so. Once again, I felt the fear stir in my belly.

I threw my will up into my mind. I had done the slopes without a protection bar, with sheer will. I would not abandon the situation, and I did not want to be abandoned by my family. I didn't go to just any bookstore; I went into the city of Boston to go to one. I headed first to the area marked "Psychology" and meandered on from there. I had so many choices. In those days I never suspected I could go wrong. I selected my reading material by following my instincts. On this day I was attracted to books related to mind over matter and behavioral response. I found myself rereading sentences, spending hours digesting only a few pages. I had studied unfamiliar subject matter before. I used a yellow highlighter, knowing I would be returning to review some of the material later. It was usually during the early-evening hours when I would sit on my bed, two pillows behind my back, with the door closed, and practice my exercise. Because I was a beginner I needed my own space and quiet time. The idea of visualization is similar to that of counting sheep when sleep won't come. Yet I not only discovered I could see the picture; I could smell it, feel it, and sense its touch as well.

I was training myself to reach higher and higher into my mind, to distract myself from my fear of the height of the mountain. I could ride the chair lift more confidently with Gordon now, opting to sit on the outside. I still preferred limited conversation, but my eyes were wide open.

Mindful of the power of visualization, I took myself to Plum Island, picturing inwardly the ocean, its massive landscape and salty smell. As I got better at visualization, my ability to evoke details became more precise. During long waits in the grocery store line, I would envision myself yodeling as I shooshed down mountains. Over the next few years I became more accomplished in my visualization. I got to a point where I could identify the number of grains in a pinch of sand. Things were beginning to change. I was taking more and more responsibility for myself. I was teaching myself to face my reality rather than live with anger, resentment, and fear.

Despite all my self-knowledge and inner work, I could be paralyzed by my father's rage during his Alzheimer years. The wild look in his eyes would cause my heart to race and my mouth to turn dry, as if I were a Boston Marathon runner approaching Heartbreak Hill. My father's fear of losing control could cause him to panic. As the situation perpetuated itself, he spun into a rage. The sequence repeated itself again and again. If he dozed off in his chair with one nurse on duty and awoke to find another standing by his chair and Mother was not there to reassure him, it was a ripe situation. Agitation did not always mean rage. It was a warning. It was saying, "You better get your ducks in order." We quieted things down. I would slow down all my movements, as well as the tone of my voice. I bored him. I talked about the ratings of the high school football team and the color of cheerleaders' costumes. It was not my job to be accurate, just to keep him distracted from seeking confrontation. If he sounded cantankerous, that was my cue to say, "Daddy, I have a dentist appointment. I will be back later." I would use the excuse of going to the dentist because I knew my father had an ingrained respect for caring for one's teeth. I purposely never gave a specific time because I knew he would read his watch. He trusted me to keep my word. I didn't want him ever to think I would stand him up.

Each shift saw his need for medication differently, and that was why monitoring his medicines was part of my daily routine. This was not a power play on my behalf but rather an act of family responsibility. The nurses all agreed. Someone needed to be in touch with the total picture. Some medicines, like Haldol, made my father worse. It was interesting to see how the same medicine could affect his behavior differently, depending on the time of day, whether he was tired or well rested, and his general degree of restlessness.

My father was not a man who liked to be touched. When a person went to take him by his hand or place their hand on his shoulder, he would jerk his arm away and thrash out in aggravation or anger. If he was addressed as "dear" he would erupt in rage. Although he never hit anyone, he came close to it. His combativeness became a family concern. Because he was too unsteady on his feet, the more experienced nurses would grab him tightly by his belt, from behind. The first time I saw this I thought the nurse was being too rough. Later I could see he felt more secure and reassured with a firm hand of authority bracing him up.

I dreaded the fear as he went out of control, so I often left the scene at his worst time. Elizabeth tells how his body would get stiff and rigid, with the resistance of an elephant. One moment he would be in a rage, the next sweet as pie. The nurses always tried to find ways to give him back his control by asking him how he felt and what he would like. While my father was in a rage, wanting his car keys, to go out for a ride, Karen pulled forth a letter she and Rhoda had concocted, signed by the governor of

Massachusetts. The document stated that people over eighty years of age were no longer able to drive. As my father was a man who lived by the law, this defused his rage, for the time being. It was really for his best well-being.

Whenever my father fell down, Gordon or John was telephoned to help get him up. God was looking out for him, because he never hit his head. A pillow placed under his head, Mother would sit by loyally. Gordon says, "Getting him up was a project. The nurse on duty would grab one arm and I would grab the other. We moved him into a sitting, then standing position. Sometimes it was easier to lift him myself, grabbing him from behind, under his armpits." It is not an unusual pattern with men to act very different with other men around. That was why when my father was enraged, strong as an elephant, his heart pounding, Gordon's presence would either snap him into being more rational or, at the very least, help him to calm down. It probably happened a dozen times: The call would come late at night. Gordon would describe to me my father's senseless speech, wild look, and loud voice, and his pacing, trying to leave the house. Especially with Gordon he would quiet down and they would talk "shop" and automobiles.

When my father was out of control he would turn his attention to me and command, "You know what to do; take care of it." Because I was unable to satisfy his demand, I became frightened and withdrawn, like a little girl. I knew I was not fooling the nurses or Mother when I treated my fear lightly by saying, "When Daddy gets angry I'm scared to death he is going to take my bike away, then send me directly to my room." We laughed, but we knew full well how frightened I truly was. That was when I got the idea of pulling from the attic some of my childhood photos and placing them among family photos, I brought downstairs some photos of Gordon as well. I had a zany impulse that Christmas of '89, to put myself on top of the tree. It was a hard Christmas. The children rolled their eyes when they entered the living room to find my eight-by-ten portrait on top of our Christmas tree, in the same location our traditional angel had sat since they were young children. The gold lettering in the corner fold told me I had sat for this portrait at Watson Studio when I was eight years old. I placed it there temporarily, just to be funny. I enjoyed giving my child self her special recognition, surrounded by lights. Whenever I passed the archway into the living room, I looked up and smiled. My family tolerated this that Christmas; they must have realized this little girl in many ways was giving me strength and insight. I had a very supportive family, yet no one was cooking my meals. I had become a superconscientious caretaker, allowing no detail of my parents' needs to get by me if I could be there for them. In my fear of letting my parents down, I had become a son and daughter all wrapped up in one, a superchild.

I developed odd habits and had strange dreams. I would half-close my eyes to find my strength, pulling my thumbs into my four fingers. I didn't indulge in cocktails, but I did more than my share of eating crackers. The snapping, brittle texture helped dull my fire so that I could think more clearly. (I didn't realize at the time, that carbohydrates are calming.) Eating one little cracker after another also helped me to take small pieces of what I had to deal with and put them in order.

One day I had a particularly silent and self-controlled morning. I had spent too many days in a row pleasing too many people with the fiber of my will. On this day I discovered a new side to my character. I took a huge deep breath and like a soldier I spit a huge gob on the lawn. It felt so releasing I concluded I had spit vim and fire in me that I had swallowed down too long. After that I became quite adept at spitting; I could see it did me good. It developed into a little ritual. I came out my back door, straightened my shoulders, sniffed the high winds, and. . . . This was the male self. I needed to balance myself up for being such a good girl. I remembered as a child seeing my father spit on occasion and thinking what a rugged, manly thing it was for such a proper man. On some level it made me feel more united with him, to think I had a habit like his, one he approved of. I remember how excited I was pulling into the driveway. I had new material to entertain them with. We were all seated at the kitchen table except for the nurse; she was standing at the kitchen sink overlooking the three of us. "Daddy" I said, "I have the best news! I have learned to spit as well as you, and best of all, it didn't take much practice." He roared with laughter and I followed, laughing so hard I nearly pulled a stitch in my side. Mother, however, sat motionless, eyes wide open, looking at me with a horrified glare. Her reaction made me laugh even harder. I thought to myself, *I know just what she's thinking: How could this crazy daughter of mine waste her time learning how to spit and then be so bold to tell us in front of the nurse. Has she no shame?* Back then I was in a three-ring circus, so to speak. I created myself as an enjoyable presence. I was going to be the caretaker in a positive, creative way of my mother or I was going to be the caretaker in a positive, creative way of my father. No matter what I did, I felt like a winner. I have never since this difficult time needed to spit. And I don't have to go into a euphoria of compulsive caretaking, either, or to be the perfect entrepreneur. I no longer apply the standards I felt I needed to uphold taking care of my family to everybody else in the world.

When I was denying the worst of what was happening in our family, intolerable fears and anxieties came to me in sleep. I must have been extremely busy in my dreams. Sometimes I was exhausted, as if I had been at death's gate during my sleep. My jaw would ache when I awoke. I tried to release this grinding grip of my will. I tried some stretching exercises, opening my mouth wide, swinging it right and left, and pulling my protruding willful jaw in. Finally I called my dentist and was fitted for a night guard. I was humiliated to think that I didn't have better control of my emotions. This plastic contraption was designed to cushion my bite, preventing me from grinding. I wore it during the worst times of my father's disease.

While I was adjusting to my father's erratic rage, Mother's nervous system was breaking down. When she did eat she had difficulty holding her food down. She would often feel chilled. Her stomach was growling all the time, a nervous reaction of many years. A woman who had always been dressed for her family before breakfast now was too weak to get dressed before noon. At the garage Eleanor was paying Mother's bills. Her trips to the hairdresser's on Thursdays were her only outside activity. There was no mystery about what was going on. It was incredibly sad and difficult to accept; my loyal, dedicated father's behavior was actually speeding my mother's dissolution.

On April 28, the day of my fifty-second birthday, Mother and I were seated in my station wagon, her hair freshly done. I decided today not to go for a ride as we usually did on Thursdays after visiting the hairdresser's. Mother was tired. The shampoo and set were getting to be too much for her. Rather than riding in the car, I sensed she needed to sit under a willow tree. I drove directly to a softly shaded neighborhood with little activity and no traffic. For two months this had been our accustomed destination when she wasn't feeling well. Seated in my blue Oldsmobile station wagon, I was glad for wide windows. The long-awaited spring sun filled the car with uncanny warmth. I remember pressing the buttons to lower the windows slightly. I wanted us to hear the bird songs. Mother needed sweet quietness. I had learned to share a daughter's love, silently.

Mother spoke first, turning her head to look straight at me. "Janet, when you drop me off at the house today I am going upstairs to bed. I'm not coming back down."

I knew immediately what she meant, and I admired her too much to ask for an explanation. "You are going to make me do it, aren't you, Mother? I am going to have to be the one to place Daddy in a nursing home."

She shook her head up and down a few times before she replied, "I can't do it; I just can't do it. He has been too good to me all his life." She gave me a stare similar to the ones she had given when I was little. Her eyes drilling into me, she said, "Janet, don't ever feel guilty about anything you have to do now for your father. We could never have come this far without you."

We sat quietly for a few more minutes. I lowered the windows farther. We could both use the fresh air. I turned the ignition on, and slowly, painstakingly, not to disturb the moment, I drove reverently round the corner and began ascending Lakeview Avenue. This allowed Mother to take in whatever struck her fancy. As we approached Eastland Terrace, I realized this had been her neighborhood for sixty-seven years. I imagined that she was think-ing how peaceful it would be to get undressed and slip between the sheets of her bed, making sure to put her electric blanket on the warmest setting.

I was very grateful that it was Thursday and Karen would be there to meet us at the back door. Of all the nurses over the past three years, Karen was the easiest to be with. She took Mother's mauve all-weather coat from her shoulders and hung it in the front hall closet. I did not want to leave my Mother's side. Luckily, my father was asleep in the living room in his gold wing back chair. I no-ticed how clean and handsome he looked, with his legs stretched out, his feet crossed and resting on the needle-point footstool. He was now wearing moccasins on days when his feet were retaining too much fluid.

Mother and I must have looked like two lost souls as we stood in the kitchen by the light switch. Karen broke the silence. Before I had a chance to mention Mother's plan, she asked, "Is everything all right?"

I spoke first, and then Mother interrupted me, say-ing, "I am going upstairs now. I'm not coming back down!"

I watched Karen's shocked expression. As a natural organizer, I grinned: "We'll refer to upstairs now as Apartment A, downstairs as Apartment B." We turned as a group, ready to ascend the landing, when I let out an uncontrollable, "Wait." Everyone stopped. "Mother," I asked, sighting my feelings, "do you have to do this on my birthday? Can't you wait one more day?"

"No," she said firmly, adding with authority, "buy yourself something from us, and be sure to make it some-thing special." Maybe she felt it was befitting to turn her household over to me on her daughter's birthday.

3

My religion is to live and die without regret.
—Milarepa, Tibetan poet and saint

Spring is a lovely time of year to die but a difficult time to mourn. I sat on the edge of my dying mother's bed watching the richly lime-colored leaves unfolding. Mother had long hinted at a deliberate death. She did not want to put my father in a nursing home any more than she wanted to go through a prolonged process of decay. The life force weakening within them both, she was ready to let life go. She only accepted food when she felt she could tolerate it.

Visiting my mother in her bedroom, I no longer ran up or took the stairs two at a time, as I had done when I was younger. Even when I was feeling hurried, I approached her in a meditative state. Sometimes I found myself imagining the stairwell as a Monet-style walking bridge connecting my parents' separate worlds. I did not want either of them to sense any urgency in my footsteps. I held onto both railings on either side of the stairwell. When my father was still sleeping upstairs, we had the second railing installed to accommodate his unsteady gait. As I climbed, placing one foot in front of the other, I would swing my shoulders back and forth the same way I did when I cross-country skied. Gearing myself up for the mystery that lay ahead, from the stairs I could look out at the tops of the trees. Living on the descending arc of life I discovered new luminosity in the leaves. I found reassurance in the constancy of nature. When I saw Mother's bedroom window opened, if only an inch, springtime and fresh air increased my sense of safety; the all-encompassing arms of Mother Nature were embracing me. Rain outside brought the sound of cleansing and purity. What must it be like for Mother to get ready to fly?

I was accustomed now to seeing from my mother's perspective. We knew that if her devoted husband had been well, he would have moved mountains to make her more comfortable. We adapted to her needs as best we could. The harsh ceiling light was seldom turned on. Until near the end, she usually sat in the purple boudoir-size wing-back chair. If she was in bed she was either lying down or sitting on the edge with her feet dangling. She got a kick out of wearing tennis socks. All of her adult life she had been asked if she was Alice Marble, the famous tennis player and champion. One day I bought tennis peds with yellow woven ribbon to replace the bobby socks she wore to bed in the winter. "You need to get with the season's fashion, Mother," I said. On the night table next to Mother's bed sat an intercom, its other half was located in the kitchen. Purchasing this simple system was the first piece of business I had done when my mother went upstairs on April 28, 1989, my birthday, to stay in touch with both needy parents. When the young nurses suggested I purchase a version commonly used in children's rooms, I quietly bucked. I had become supersensitive to people regarding the elderly as children, I chose a more adult monitor system.

One day a nurse placed the piano seat between the two beds in Mother's room, because it was less obstructive than a chair. My mother had been a soloist at the Saint James Church at the age of thirteen. In later years, during holiday celebrations she would sing her favorite tunes, like "Galway Bay" and "Oh, What a Beautiful Morning" while her friend Hap played the piano. I liked sitting on the bench with her favorite sheet of music beneath me. Later I took the same music with me to the Alzheimer unit.

Not since my childhood had I explored the upstairs so thoroughly. As a child I had been a snooper of keen observation. Now when Mother was being tended to I would meander around the upstairs and sadly take in the subtle changes. Though my bedroom had been turned into a sitting room, detailed memories, full of feeling, came to me, like the warm stillness of falling asleep surrounded by the glow of Christmas candles in the windows. I rocked myself side to side like a baby and smiled to see Mother's size 5 shoes lined up perfectly along the bottom shelf of my closet, which once had held shoe boxes filled to the brim with my movie star collection. In 1951 my father had built a small bathroom off their bedroom. Mother liked to be in fashion but was not a supporter of change when it came to her daily routine and continued to use the bath at the end of the hall, the same one my sister and I shared. I liked the full-sized closet in her bathroom best of all. It smelled as I always remembered it, with a mixture of facial cream, polish remover, and witch hazel.

Each time this journey downstairs to face the complexities of my father's Alzheimer's disease filled me with fear and anxiety. There were times I experienced the stairway as a bridge to the subconscious: the black-shingled cellar roof partially cut off my view to the outside world. I would tiptoe quietly, hoping the sound of my footsteps would not trigger his deep-seated concern for his wife. When she was on his mind his level of frustration could turn the whole household upside down. Sneak-

101

ing around him was not a pleasant feeling, yet the sidesteps I took were for his sake. I would exit the house from the farthest door from where he was sitting, then walk around the house and in the other door. This strategy served many purposes. On most days my parents had very different needs and I needed time to pause and shift gears.

I always wanted to give my father my very best. My gifts for drama emerged forth fully under the stress of these times. My father was enjoying my productions. I had never before performed for my father alone. I hoped my mother was relieved to hear my father's laughter sounding up the stairwell. She could roll over comfortably now and rest from the responsibilities she had been carrying for so long. If my father's confusion intensified with worry about my mother, his eyes would dilate into a wide-eyed stare. His sentences now had become shorter. Although he lacked clarity in his ordinary communications, I assumed that he could understand me on other levels. I remember my mother-in-law, when she was active as a private duty nurse, telling how upset she would be to hear family members speaking to one another in the presence of an unconscious patient as though the person were already dead. My reading about different levels of the mind also led me to believe there was a real possibility my father knew in some ways what was going on. His intuitive behavior further led me to give him the benefit of the doubt. I noticed that when other people did not share my beliefs, rather than entertaining him, they would tend to amuse themselves. They talked about politics because politics interested them. They would speak in generalities on neutral ground to distract themselves from the realities of his illness.

As my mother's life forces waned, our children

wanted private and intimate communication with their grandparents. They would sometimes ask a nurse to leave the room if she was shadowing their visit. It was reassuring for me to see how comfortable and inventive they were in taking control. Our daughter Cindy tells of the day she was sitting at the foot of the bed watching her grandmother's motionless body curled up, facing the wall. Wanting to bring spirit and life to the moment, finally she spoke: "Grammie, I have a secret to tell you, but you cannot tell anyone. You are the first person to know." Pausing to build intrigue she added, "Do you want to hear?"

Unable to resist a juicy piece of news, my mother rolled over, looked Cindy straight in the eye, and said, "What is it?" I can only imagine the special bond they shared when Cindy replied, "Grammie, "I'm pregnant."

Mother had been upstairs and out of sight now for four days; Father was trying to fathom why. It was Saturday, May 1, Kentucky Derby Day. Elizabeth was feeling sorry for him. He was a man who had always been happiest at work. Saturdays were hard for him. He was no longer going to the country club to golf or play cards. That afternoon Elizabeth, with a strong passion to alleviate my father's sorrow, coaxed my mother to get dressed and go downstairs to join him. "Ted's lonely, Alice," she said. "He needs to be with you. We'll have our usual Saturday night happy hour, popcorn included, in the family room, and dinner as well. Ted likes that." My parents had always taken an interest in popular sports events. Mother enjoyed the clothes and the wide-brimmed hats of the Kentucky Derby. Elizabeth enjoyed the annual race in her way, too. On this late afternoon lined up in front of the tube, each chose a horse. My father, in his most quizzical tone, turned to Elizabeth and asked, "Which horse did you say you took?" When she told him, he answered, "That's the same one I chose." Following the other person's lead was how my father wrapped himself in appropriateness. Later on when he was a resident at the Alzheimer unit I noticed other patients using the same technique.

The excitement of the Derby grew as the traditional tunes sounded from the television. Elizabeth tells how she was the first to chime in: "The corn-top's ripe and the mead-ow's in the bloom, While the birds make mu-sic all the day"; Mother, in a poignant voice, followed: "Then Weep no more, my lady, Oh! weep no more today!" To everyone's surprise, my father, who never sang in church or at football games, joined in missing not a word. "We will sing one song for the old Kentucky home, For the old Kentucky home, far-a-way." That special afternoon I remembered running with my sister across our backyard to hang on doorknobs May baskets, handmade out of soft crepe paper and dancing around Maypoles. Now on May 1 I think of my parents and Elizabeth and how grateful I am that their final day together, downstairs as a couple, ended on such a musical note.

My mother had been back and forth at death's door for three years, and my father had been diagnosed with Alzheimer's for approximately the same length of time. It was not unusual for me to lie in bed at night and ask myself which parent could live better without the other? It never occurred to me I would be part of that decision until Elizabeth, the nurse, said to me over the phone one Sunday evening, "You and Barbara may want to place a 'no code' on your mother." She explained that as a result, should either parent become seriously ill no extraordinary measures would be taken to keep him or her from death. "You have the order placed with the nurses' notes; it usually goes in the front of the book. As long as you are thinking in terms of 'no code,' you may want to give consideration to your father as well." My sister and I felt confident our parents wanted natural deaths. Mother implied this the day she went upstairs. Her philosophy regarding old age had not changed over the years. She was still reiterating, "By the time you're old you've either done everything you want to do or else it's too late. You like seeing the grandchildren, but for the most part life is over."

My father, however, saw life as a very special gift, accepting all its warts. He was not one to seek a perfect world or to circumvent decay. However, he was a man who could not tolerate confinement. The thought of wearing a seat belt in his automobile or having his bed covers tucked in drove him mad. How could my father at eighty-eight years of age, unable to reason and unable to follow direction, tolerate being confined to bed? On May 19, 1989, my sister and I placed a "no code" order on both our parents.

One day I realized that the nursing service was not keeping new nurses up-to-date and informed about the "no code" policy. Privately I fumed and decided to spot-check the nurses myself, weekly on all three shifts. Not particularly diplomatic, I spoke directly to them: "Have you seen the 'no code' sheet in the front of the book?"

While we were fighting to support my mother's wishes to die according to her terms, several of the nurses wanted me to convince Mother to change her attitude and to rally. I did not want the nurses to see just how arrogantly I thought they were behaving. I knew they had good intentions. Five years previously I had been privileged to take a medical ethics course with Dr. Peggy

Walsh, who had received the Christian A. Johnson Chair Award in Ethics and Values. I remember how proud I felt to have been one of her students when I read the write-up in *Time* magazine. What I had learned about the right to die in her class told me what my sister and I were doing was clearly moral.

One day Andrea, the three-to-eleven nurse, motioned me into the upstairs sitting room for a "one-on-one" conversation. She was a registered nurse as well as a hospice volunteer and I held her knowledge and her perspective in high regard. She spoke right to the point: "Your Mother does not have to die, you know. We can have a tube inserted into her abdomen and feed her that way." I could feel my eyes narrowing as Andrea placed the tip of her index finger against her side, indicating where the incision would be made. I thought of my mother's sixty-two-pound body. I said nothing. I hoped Andrea would choke on her own words. She continued, in a professional tone, "It is a small surgical procedure and we can have it done right here at home."

There was a long pause. I allowed myself ample time to gather my thoughts and to play my strategy. I tended to talk too much when I was anxious. I worked hard keeping my face expressionless, the same way I imagined my father and his friends did when they played poker. Our swords had crossed. There were some battles I would not lose. This would be one. Because I knew my mother's mind I knew she wanted to die under her own volition. Countless times I had heard her say, "Life has come down to going to the hairdresser's on Thursday. This is not living." And now, when I thought of her in her bed, full of life in her choice to die, determined to ask in my most motherly tone, "Andrea, are you having difficulty letting go? If you are, I understand." I thought of my friend Nick and

went on, "I have a close doctor friend, a seasoned oral surgeon. He told me once how frustrating his line of work
could be doing everything possible to save a tooth, knowing ultimately it will need to be pulled. I also know you
lost a seven-year-old nephew last year. Is this a part of
your desire not to let my mother move on?"

I was astonished by her response: "What is going on
here is wrong, and that is why I called the doctor's office
the other day and told them so." The judgmental tone in
her voice told me she believed we were treating my
mother inappropriately by letting her eat only when she
wanted to and when she thought her body could tolerate
the food. I was angry Andrea had called the doctor's office
but even angrier with her arrogance.

If Andrea was showing anxiety accepting my
mother's concept of a quietly fading death, in a congenial,
familiar setting, I wondered whether other nurses were
feeling apprehensive as well. What was needed was open
dialogue. The following morning I called the doctor's office and requested a house call. Mr. Hogan had been to
our house in the early days of Mother's recovery and
when my father was recovering from his prostate surgery. An older gentleman, I was sure he had given
thought to his own death.

As I sat patiently in the upstairs den waiting to hear
the report, my thoughts wandered downstairs, to my father, dozing in his chair. I stood to greet Mr. Hogan. I saw
kindness in his eyes as he said, "I will order a oxygen tank
to be delivered tomorrow. Your mother may be needing it
later. It will help to make her more comfortable."

I thought oxygen tanks were for people who had difficulty breathing. *Does it hurt to die?* I wondered. I spoke
directly and simply because I wanted to say it only once:
"Mr. Hogan, do you know what we are trying to do here?"

He looked straight into my eyes, nodded his head slightly, and with a half-smile said, "This is what your mother wants and the family is doing a good job."

I wanted the major issues out in the open. I continued, "Some of the nurses are having difficulty in accepting the family wishes."

He nodded. He repeated one more time. "The family is doing a good job." The words *case closed* quietly glided beyond me, like a colorful hot air balloons at a festival.

Yet it was Andrea, who had objected most dramatically to Mother's mode of dying, who taught me, with her hospice experience, not to be afraid of mentioning the Hereafter in front of my mother. After Mother had died I offered Andrea the Swiss music box she had brought upstairs and placed on the lamp table across from the foot of my mother's bed. Its soft miniature music had filled the room with serenity.

Every night I thought this would be the night, yet Mother was still there the next morning. I had no idea it took so long to die. We maintained special foods for special times of the day, keeping odors in the house that would make her happy, like the smell of home-baked beans or freshly baked apple. We gently encouraged her to eat but did not force her. The plate shrank, getting smaller and smaller, until her nutrients fit in a custard cup.

Though I had grown up in a house with few religious rituals, I had been well guided by high standards. Because I was raised in a place of safe nesting, my mind was free to fly, to look for mystery in the beyond. My father had asked me when I was in my early teens, "Why do you send for religious books? I didn't teach you to do that!" From a monthly book club I had ordered books by religious writers, like the Reverend Billy Graham, the Reverend Peter Marshall, and Norman Vincent Peale. It was not my intention to read each book cover to cover. As a teenager I was looking for stories in which people overcame struggle. As I look back now, I can see that I was trying to find neutral ground within my parents' different religious backgrounds. As I introduced myself to spirituality, I learned that the road to life is full of bumps and curves. I discovered that nevertheless there is a spiritual force within and beyond. Downstairs in the playroom, at eight o'clock in the evening, after my father had finished playing pool, I let it all out. With great gusto I sang songs full of spirit that I had learned in Sunday school and patriotic songs, similar to those you would hear at a parade, my portable record player providing my accompaniment. It was here my mind took flight regarding religion and the beyond. In my youth I was not a "goody-goody" regarding religion. I always made it work to my benefit. My spiritual beliefs instilled in me a strong sense of confidence and forgiveness. They allowed me to be courageous and bold. With great delight I participated in popular church school pranks. I recall Sunday mornings my mother placing my church offering envelope on the dining room table. My father enclosed the fifty-cent piece, and I licked the flap before placing the envelope into my purse. When my sister and I were dropped off at the front of the church for Sunday school, she would go inside while I crossed over to the opposite corner, joining my friends at the soda fountain. Max, the owner, exchanged our half-dollars for two quarters, one for God and one for ourselves.

Not until I was married myself did I notice how consistent my parents had been in accommodating each other. My father would never think to be late without calling; my mother never kept him waiting. My mother had grown up Catholic; for his sake as a parent she took on the role of good Protestant, a supportive nonactive member. My father had a special relationship to the Catholic Church. You heard a proud chuckle when he boasted how he had donated pulpits to three Catholic churches. He enjoyed priests and frankly respected their salesmanship; as an automobile dealer he was interested in the practical details of the building up of a church. It was my mother's choice to have my sister and me raised as Protestants.

My mother was not a person to do things halfway. Each Sunday, Barbara and I would be dressed to the "tens" in hand-smocked dresses, and patent-leather shoes. We were always appareled in colors appropriate to the season, our hair adorned with bows that my mother had made from specially chosen ribbon. My father drove us to Protestant Sunday school weekly but only accompanied us to church for holidays and special services. I remember my mother joining us only once for a special children's pageant. Whenever I asked about her absence, she would reply, "I have a one-thirty dinner to cook, vegetables to peel, a roast to put in the oven, plus a pie to make." When I was older I would wonder why she did not cook a steak or add pie to her weekly bakery order. Even though my mother did not accompany us to church, I knew she was not without religious rituals of her own. On rare occasions when I was asked to make up my mother's bed, I found crystal rosary beads tucked under her pillow. As a child I liked to pick them up and act out being holy, resting them solemnly in both my hands and mumbling godly, as I had seen my Catholic friends do when we attended Good Friday services together. Sometimes, as I walked through the door on my return home from church,

110

I would hear organ music and hymns coming from the radio. I would wonder whether she had listened to this while we were gone or just turned the radio on to hear the twelve o'clock news, but I never asked her. I now realize how careful my mother was not to let religion intrude on her relationship to the man she loved. They did not banter lightly about significant matters; peace had been her priority.

While my mother was working at putting her house in order, Elizabeth, the nurse, helped to put Mother's spirituality in order. As a former nun, Elizabeth knew the language of the church. She could address the Catholic part of my mother. Because she was a Catholic girl who had been excommunicated by her own volition I wondered if it was appropriate to request a priest to come to the house to give her the Last Rites. I sensed his visit would feel awkward to her. I knew my mother was not afraid to die. Elizabeth told me, "I spent a long time asking your mother if she had any fears. We spoke about familiarizing yourself with death and then you have nothing to fear." I wish I could have been less tired and preoccupied with my father. I would have been dependent on nurses and opened my heart more fully to my dying mother so we could have spoken honestly about impermanence. I wish I had been less shy about lighting candles and introducing prayer into our visits.

My mother always had been a modest and unassuming woman. She was not looking for a death full of fanfare and celebration. What she wanted most was peace and quiet. Being upstairs was more tranquil for her. I admired her courage. Now, looking back, I am able to see her strength was not merely courage; it was more part of her authentic self. She graciously accepted what she was. She did not totally give up, but she did not exercise heroics. When she was up to conversing, she did; otherwise she settled into the silence. If anybody is ever ready to die, she was ready. In the depths of her soul she had named her fear: she was more afraid of the Alzheimer's than she was of death.

As a family we were learning how to balance the quality of care given to my parents. As an Alzheimer patient my father had a pace of his own. If you tried to rush him he would resist. My mother needed assistance to motivate herself or she showed signs of decline. The idea of day care came to mind, if only a few hours of the day, preferably mornings. I scheduled a return visit with Wendy, the home care coordinator at the hospital. She informed me that part-time day care services were available. I knew that was for us. Yet as I was driving my car across town to the facility, a new, unexpected, and somewhat vain concern came over me. How would my father be received—not by the patients themselves but by their family members and friends? The day-care facility was an extension of the nursing home located less than a mile from my parents' house. Standing in the center of the activity room, I looked around with an approving eye. I said to the administrator, "Our family is in a life-and-death situation. We need to have this center as a daily option for an unknown length of time, as soon as possible. Yesterday would not be too soon."

I was taken aback by the injustice in what she said: "If the family takes responsibility for the cost, your father can start tomorrow morning, eight until noon; otherwise, you will need to wait ten days. It takes that long for health insurance papers to be processed." I swallowed my rage at the inequity of it, but I saw the practical side. His money again could be used to support his dignity and my mother's. Karen, the nurse, liked to call it the Club (in reference to the country club my father had formerly attended). My father went along with the jibe, reluctantly! Always a punctual man, now he leaned toward lateness. Gordon drove him there. After these trips, I heard Gordon often say, "Dropping your father off broke my heart." Yet it brought peace at home. To ensure a smooth transition, Karen went along for the ride, not only for my father but to instruct the care takers as well. My father had always been his own boss. He was not accustomed to being told what to do. Karen was a pro at letting him think everything was his idea.

We were disappointed that my father was not happy at his new club, a situation beyond our control. Whenever Gordon went to pick him up my father would say as he stepped into the car, "The people around here are crazy." He never participated in the activities, but he was charming and did what he was asked. He came home tired and ready to nap. Acting appropriately can be hard work, particularly when your mind is against you. By the second week, he was hollering, "Get me home!" and insisted on making a phone call.

I purchased a vest restrainer and put it in the lower drawer of the dining room credenza. Now for sure we had to hire nurses upstairs and down, especially for him, an expensive proposition, but we were going for broke. It was his earnings taking care of him, and this was what we wanted, too. Friends and acquaintances looked upon us as being extravagant and foolish. It stirred up my whole value system when I heard respected members of the community saying, "I hope my children never spend my hard-earned money so recklessly." I was reassured by my father's extraordinary honesty and years and years of good deeds. Fortunately, I felt relatively secure, and I did not need my parents' money. Nor did my sister. Night nurses, daytime nurses, upstairs nurses, and downstairs nurses gave us freedom of choice and peace of mind.

My father always had a simple, straightforward, honest relationship with his money. He had been working since he was eleven years old, and he was proud of his money, like any self-made person. Something very fundamental within him said, *I've got to take care of myself.* Today, at the turn of the new century, people in his situation would take a more sophisticated approach with their hard-earned money. With communications and the level of information that is available, it's hard to be simple with money anymore. But my father knew how much money his sons-in-law earned, and he knew his daughters were taken care of very well and his grandchildren also were going to be well cared for through their own competence. He didn't feel obliged to give them money, even though he was a very generous man.

I recall my mother telling stories she'd heard while vacationing in Florida of sad, angry parents who had turned over their estates to their children with an agreement that they would still be taken care of, only to have the children take the money and spend it on themselves.

My sister and I had as simple and straightforward a philosophy toward my father's money as he did. We wished to do for him what we knew he would for his wife. It was his money and not yet our inheritance. It was our belief that a good portion of the money we were spending would otherwise go to Uncle Sam, so why not spend it lavishly on him? Maybe this was unusual that the family all agreed, but we did. Every now and again I would check in with Eleanor, my father's bookkeeper, and ask, "Is it time to consider an alternate plan?" She knew I wanted two years' advance notice if we were beginning to run low. She usually answered with a comment like, "No, but we'll keep an eye on it." We were aware the money was dwindling and that we might eventually spend his entire estate.

The regular nurses accommodated us by working additional shifts. We had few newcomers, yet one came well recommended from the nursing service. I was upstairs with my mother seated in her bedroom chair. Mother was in bed with her face turned to the wall. I assumed she was sleeping. The girl came into the room and carelessly plunked herself at the foot of my mother's bed without glancing Mother's way. This young whipper-snapper of a nurse proceeded to say, "I don't know how you can stand it."

I said, "What do you mean?"

She continued, "Your father. How did you stand it all those years growing up in the same house with that stubborn man?"

"What is giving you so much difficulty?" I asked. I had trouble connecting the word *stubborn* with my father. As I saw it, he had a long history of strong will that allowed her and the other nurses to be here.

"He doesn't want to give me his teeth. His bridge is to come out at night. He doesn't want to give it to me."

Straining to keep my cool, I said, "He only has control over giving you his bridge; he doesn't even have control over his bladder anymore. All he is saying to you is that he wants a little bit of control in his life. Maybe he knows it's still daylight and early. Does it really matter to you whether or not you have, now, his bridge in your hand?"

Looking somewhat sheepish, she said, "Well, if you put it like that, I guess not."

I said, "Why don't you go for a walk? It's lovely outside, one can tire of being in the house."

She said, "Really?"

And I said, "Yes, be gone thirty or thirty five minutes. It's fine with me. Go around the block a couple of times if you'd like."

My grown nephew John Junior was there at the time. He knew my dander was up. And he said, "Auntie, you are bad." I smiled and proceeded to call the nursing service to send a different nurse the following day.

Although I had a household budget, I was not financially adept. Women investment clubs had not yet emerged. I had done much, but I had not earned an income. Many of my decisions about money were unconscious; what I simply wanted was to get the job done, I had been brought up to leave financial aspects to the men.

I recalled a church council meeting in the late 1980s. I held the position of chairman of the Long-Range Planning Committee. I had just finished giving the committee report. Al, the church treasurer, looked over at me, with a crooked smile, his eyebrows raised. "Janet," he said, "every time you get on a committee it costs the church money."

"Al," I replied, "just keep it coming; we have a lot of work to get done."

I was gradually learning to take more complete charge of both my father and my mother. I was the self-appointed functioning substitute matriarch of the family. I orchestrated special "calling hours," for Mother's Day. In retrospect, I can see how planning these events was my way of releasing built-up tension. I found it exhilarating, like a good run or an advanced step-aerobic class. The other family members seemed to have much less capacity to engage in these caregiving activities. It was my plan, that day, to empower and involve others so that my mother, at the end of the day, could return to her bed with fresh, updated conversations dancing in her head until the end of her time. I asked people to jockey around their holiday schedules to accommodate this special day and to drop by one or two at a time, a reasonable number for Mother.

Like any overly zealous daughter, I wanted my mother meticulously dressed for this special, final Mother's Day. Her grandmother-of-the-bride dress I thought would do fine, the one she planned to be laid out in. Mother insisted a nightgown with her bed jacket would be "good enough." I returned to the local store where, as a child, I had heard my mother order her underwear over the phone and where, three years previous, she had sent me to buy her two bed jackets. Mother had always preferred quilted bathrobes, and now especially I could see why. (Mother never bought one of anything. She always thought in terms of "extras, just in case.") I described my mother's needs. A gray-haired middle-aged woman came out of the back room carrying two drab, limp jackets. I selected a quilted bedjacket. It puffed her up a bit in all the right places. I did not intend to treat my mother as a dying old lady. I realized I was free to buy bows with sequins and polka dots. I had my mother's spunk and spirit. She chose to sit wearing it in her purple wingback chair. She agreed to have her hair touched up, lipstick freshly applied, in order to greet each family member one at a time.

I knew my mother was used to my shenanigans. Whenever I got cranked up, like I was on this particular day, Mother would just sit back, take it all in, and permit me to carry on until I ran out of gas. There were times I can imagine her saying, "If you'd just go home, child, and leave me alone, I might be able to get on with my dying." As I took the gown from the hanger in the back of the closet, I said, "Tomorrow, Mother, you can wear this ice blue one, the one we bought three years ago when you were in the hospital. The satin still has a sheen and looks like new. These appliqued butterflies across the top make me think of spring. It may not match like a bride's peignoir," (her eyes rolled back in her head), "but it will coordinate well with your pink quilted bed jacket. Oh, by the way, Mother, keep the top button closed and the rest opened. It looks more casual that way. And don't forget to wear your round pearl earrings. They match that very same button."

Mother replied with a smile on her face and a flip of her wrist, "Get out of here! Go home to your family where you belong." As I look back now, I can see that I was holding back my sorrow and grief by being extraordinarily absorbed in detail.

It was six o'clock on Mother's Day evening. I was home impatiently twiddling my thumbs, wondering how Mother's "calling hours" were going. *Tomorrow she will be too tired to talk,* I thought. I imagined my father was asleep in his chair, all the excitement and comings and goings have worn him out and the cookie jar our son, Jeff, had filled the day before empty. I would not be surprised to see Mother's face pale and her eyes drawn, after greeting twelve people. When I arrived later I flopped myself at the end of what once had been my father's twin bed. Seated directly across from her, I was able to pick up on each gleam in her eye. She surprised me by saying, "Where have you been? When you didn't show up I began to worry." In my euphoria of service, I had forgotten to tell her why I stayed away. I realized I was making decisions

118

in my mother's behalf while at the same time leaving her in the dark.

One day I blew my stack. My anger was directed at Mother. For well over a week she had been up and down, mostly down. You could hear it in the nurse's voices when they gave their reports. Her robe had not been taken off the hanger for days, and the oxygen tank was by her bed. From the top of the upstairs landing I could see her in bed, half-comatose or weakly seated upright in her chair. One afternoon I found her neither in bed nor in her chair. I walked from room to room weaving in and out of control, "Mother, where are you? Where have you gone? It is bad enough I come here every day not knowing what I will find. Where have you disappeared to? You have me on a roller-coaster ride. You know I never liked roller-coasters as a child."

Her voice came from the left a short distance down the hall. "Janet, calm down," she said. "What's gotten into you? I am here in the john, sitting on the throne."

As a parent of three I had experiences as an authority figure, yet I had never laid down the law to my mother. I was surprised one day to hear myself being harsh with her. It was no secret that one reason my mother had gone upstairs was to separate herself from my father's Alzheimer behavior. At eighty-nine years of age she was frail, weighing in at sixty-two pounds; her nervous system was shattered and breaking down. What I found cruel and unacceptable was her completely turning her back on him. Knowing how devoted he had been to her for sixty-nine years, I didn't know how else to say it. I just spit it out. "Mother," I said, "Daddy is a very decent man and deserves more from you more than what you are giving. He is worthy of a daily visit. This is nonnegotiable. You and the nurses set the time of day!"

The visits began. To prepare him, the nurses fussed like they might have with a young son going off on a special date. They combed his hair, moisturized his face, and removed the breakfast spots on his sweater. As it turned out, the visits went more smoothly than did his journey up and down the stairs. The nurses held onto his sturdy leather belt from behind. The return trip back downstairs was awkward and sometimes dangerous. I was reminded of an expression my father oftentimes used when describing his good fortune: "The harder I work, the luckier I get."

My father had always been a direct and insightful man. It was not unusual to hear him say when someone at the dealership had to be let go and no one wanted to do it, "You can't run a business from your heart; it has to come from your head." One Sunday afternoon Elizabeth reported to me this poignant conversation. It was so moving I wrote it down in my journal.

"Hi, Al. How are you doing?"

"OK, Ted."

"Anything I can get you?"

"No, Ted."

"Do you need a new dress?"

"No," as she rolled her eyes and tilted her head down to her bathrobe.

"That's right, that's right," he said. "Maybe I can get you a new bathrobe. Want a new bathrobe?"

"No, I'm all set, Ted. I'm all set."

"Is there anything at all you want, Al?"

"No, Ted. There's nothing at all."

"Is there anyplace you want to go, Al?"

"No, Ted. There's no place I want to go. Is there anyplace that you would like to go, Ted?"

"No, I've seen it all. Well, I've seen everything I wanted to see. Is there anything you want to do, Al?"

"No, Ted. There's nothing I want to do. Is there anything you want to do, Ted?"

"No. I did everything I wanted to do. I've seen everything I wanted to see. I'm very satisfied, Al. Al, are you satisfied?"

"Yes, Ted. I'm satisfied."

"Al, what do I do now?"

"You go downstairs, Ted. You go downstairs. Sit in your chair. Be quiet and wait."

Today I am able to see underneath my anxiety about living without regrets and why fear had me running around in circles. In the beginning of my parents' illnesses I subconsciously saw my caretaker position as an opportunity to repent for times in my childhood when I had unknowingly and knowingly disappointed both parents. I needed to repent for not having been a boy. I was my father's final chance to have a son. When I was born they did not even have a girl's name picked out. My father wanted to name me Aldana, a combination of both their names, Alice and Dana, but my mother did not go along with that. Four days later, after they agreed on the name Janet, a nurse at the desk filling out a form asked my father, "What is your daughter's middle name to be?"

My father replied, "Forget the middle name—it took us four days to come up with the first."

As "son," and daughter, I wanted to carry out all their desires perfectly. I wanted my mother to die according to her wishes.

Teetering on the edge of life, Mother sprang onward like the Eternal Fountain of Hope. I drank gulps of optimism against all reason, returning again and again to the house. I knew my enthusiasm, at full tilt, could knock the pins out from anyone with declining energy. Especially on Mother's good days I tried to harness my joy until in my car I would hoot out at the top of my lungs, "Yippee! Yippee! Thank You! Thank You, Lord, for giving us one more time." Back then I saw life in increments of hours.

I respected Mother's painstaking effort to organize her death. Even when she was tired of the business of homemaking, she put her whole self into it. And now I was trying to keep up with this little Irish wild woman with such tremendous sense of responsibility, my father lurking unpredictable in the shadows, one moment sweet, the next a tyrant. There were mornings when I went to visit, just days before she died, she had the night nurse write a list: "Vanity Fair napkins, Vaseline Intensive Care." She was still thinking in terms of caring for her husband. Another note stated: "Bring your father's portrait down from the attic and have it hung in the dealership after everything has quieted down." I believe my mother expected my father to be placed in a nursing home shortly after she died, unable to imagine her Alzheimer husband remaining at home without her care. How was she to know that without the stress of a dying wife, my father's condition would change, that for a while he would become less frustrated and more manageable?

There were days I found I was unable to inhale a deep breath. Like my mother, who once carried smelling salts in her pocketbook, I now carried a doctor's prescribed inhaler. If I couldn't keep my own emotions in line how was I to assist others? I was ashamed of needing any kind of help. As I stood at the pharmacy counter, waiting for my inhaler, I checked out the vitamin display. Because I did not want to be reminded of my shortcomings every time I opened my purse, I placed the inhaler and B vitamins in a small cosmetic pouch out of my sight. In my extreme feeling of responsibility for all concerned, I had one fear greater than all the other fears, and it swirled around in my head like steam. What if by chance some warm spring morning my Alzheimer father awakes and, because he feels like himself, he climbs the stairs alone and disoriented, visits his wife, and finds she is dying? What will I say if he turns to me and asks, "Janet, how could you have let this happen?"

My sister had given me permission early on to take on added responsibility. I not only took it on; I also tried to be three children (the "Son") wrapped up in one. All this dutiful, inventive helpfulness was making me a little bit crazy. I was in a euphoria of service being the entertainer, the loving one, the organizer, the one who's there all the time, the one whose parents are her primary responsibility, hiring nurses, watching over all the details, day after day after day, month after month, year after year suppressing my grief and my rage. I can see more clearly now how underneath the drive to please, to be the best possible caretaking daughter for them, was a tremendous helpless, childish fear. Had I done enough? Had I lived up to their high standards? Was I deserving of their love? I feared that if I did not give 110 percent and "do it right" the feeling of letting my parents down would wipe me out. From the time I was a child I was schooled in pleasing these two different people, but never did I attempt with more determination and consciousness than when they were sick and dying.

There were times when I feared my body was breaking down. Now and again, when I was visiting my parents, one of them would notice and comment, "You're not walking quite right; what's bothering you?"

I liked having a few standard answers. "Nothing," I said. "Just my Achilles tendon tightening up." During the day it ached and felt stiff; at night it burned like fury. Some nights when I crawled into bed my body felt like a live lobster laid flat on the fisherman's slab and sliced down the center to be "baked stuffed." I would lie in bed and recall Fridays at Herb's Fish Market, watching, with fascination, the process. One day while watching Donald slice a sea urchin open, I asked, "Is he dead?"

"What do you think? Wouldn't you be if I did that to you?"

With a scrunched-up face and eyes wide opened, I asked, "Well, why is he still moving?"

Donald shook his head, shrugged his shoulders, and walked off.

When I returned, the following Friday, I worked my way around to the subject of lobsters, asking, "Was that movement his nerve endings responding?"

"You got it, lady." Donald said. "You got yourself a gold star."

Little did he know at home in my top desk drawer I had several small sheets of gold stars. Some I kept for myself, and others I included in birthday cards.

I changed the vivid image of a prepared lobster and envisioned my body filled with healing salt from the sea, with large ocean sponges absorbing the sting as they delicately patted the open cavity. Resolved to take good care of myself, I gave time to visualizing and tending to my own body's needs. I had learned that from my father. As a young man, newly in business, each month he had gone to Harry Hershfield, his podiatrist, and had him "work on" his feet. I would hear my father say, "If my feet aren't healthy, I'm out of business."

My parents' home was now a full house, and I was

afraid that if I relaxed for one minute, the whole house of cards would come tumbling down. "Ask Janet," had become the family battle cry. I found I was defending myself against the curiosity of other family members who were not so involved. Because I was in such an intense mode of responsibility and attention, anyone's questions could put me into a tailspin. I did not have extra energy to keep explaining things to everybody. I felt that it was too hard for them to really grasp what was happening in the strange communications setup, and so I found myself defending myself against their curiosity and potential judgment of my behavior, even if their curiosity was kindly and candid. Barbara and I had agreed not to speak daily. I was at fever pitch. I was praying like a crazy woman. My parents were dying and I was on the edge. I was so fired up and my sense of responsibility was so wide that I couldn't relate to cool inquirers. Now I can see I was so wound up I was difficult to approach. I desperately needed to be the one in charge. On a difficult day when I was especially feeling my father's neediness, I was acutely sensitive to the ignorance and misunderstanding of others who were not so close to the situation and yet were trying to tell me what to do. When you are hard pressed it is easier to do it yourself.

Some days I wondered if taking care of my parents was going to turn me into an old lady before my time. My role was causing me to take on more weight, and this was a concern. I knew how the body compensates during distressing circumstances. Some people get bone thin; instead, I was holding on by plumping up and cushioning myself. There were days I was on the edge of insanity, grasping for straws. I knew my body was out of balance when I started to crave sweets, a reflection of the bitter situation. I never bought more than one candy bar at a time. But many a night I drove to the corner store, under the pretense of doing an errand, and returned home only after satisfying my newly acquired sweet tooth, or I would run out to get a book to lift me up and fill me with sanity. I always bought two rather than one. I gave the second book away to anyone who appeared interested in the subject, hoping to surround myself with people who would think the same way I did. More than anything else I wanted to be understood, not misinterpreted, because I was energetically bigger and stronger than most. In tense situations, rather than pull back, I pushed myself to go beyond, hoping I would then produce a better situation. The bull rises within me and I take the horns of the bull *and* the tail; I can feel my cosmic tail swishing. I have watched people stand around waiting for me so they can ride on my tail. I am accustomed to it, but I get angry about it. I have often wished for people to show more initiative. Sometimes I am envious of them, and yet this is the way I am.

My parents' bedroom, which we were now calling Mother's room, had been fashionable but not luxurious thirty years ago. I recall how proud Mother had been with her choice of bright colors: purple, off white, and royal blue. Her bed was located to the right up against the outside wall. A nightstand separated the twin beds. A radio, simple alarm clock, and crystal lamp sat on the table, along with a intercom. Since my sister and I had moved from the house Mother had been using other bedroom closets. The piano bench placed along the side of my mother's bed gave me a sense of freedom of movement. I could be close yet slip out without having to disturb her. I was always aware that I did not want to take air from her or interfere with her view out the window. I was in a musical situation and I needed to play the composition by ear, to be spontaneous and careful and subtle in my expression.

When Elizabeth, the nurse, suggested Barbara and I make arrangements at the funeral home ahead of time rather than waiting until "it happens," I thought, *This is my kind of lady.* Elizabeth added, "Rather than running around the day it happens, by planning ahead you can take a bubble bath instead." Barbara and I had never taken part in arranging a funeral before. We met in the parking lot of the funeral home and went to the back entrance together. I was nervous, as much for my sister as for myself. I was in my tending-to-all-possible-details mode; like my father, I was anxious to keep the books clean and to be proud at the end of the day. Barbara was visibly shaken and said she wanted this meeting over with as quickly as possible. We both agreed doing it ahead of time would be much easier than later on. When it was time to plan the Memorial Obituary, it was nice not having to do it alone. I never realized my mother was vain regarding her age until Barbara said, "Don't include what year she was born." We were reassured by the director that the funeral would be private and at the family's convenience. We decided to have memorial contributions made to a charity of the donor's choice.

I was taken aback when the funeral director motioned for us to follow him. I had no idea we would be selecting a coffin right off a display room floor. Somehow I thought we would choose from photographs in a three-ring binder, like purchasing telegraph flowers from a florist. As we entered the large display room, the coffins were arranged like automobiles in a showroom, allowing members of the family to walk up close, touch them, even look inside. I was distracted by the wall covering, the same scenic paper Mother had chosen for her dining room, years back. I saw my sister also was spooked by the ordeal when I asked if she wanted to step out for a moment and she said, "No, I want to do this." I noticed to the left of the entranceway was a coatrack filled with dresses, men's sports coats, shirts, and ties. I was told these were extra garments made available to people who had been residing in rest homes and for the convenience of families who were from out of town and did not wish to shop. Barbara suggested we narrow our choices by selecting the coffin that we believed would be my father's choice. Five minutes later we were ready to leave. The director asked us to drop off at our convenience a hymnal marked with songs we would like to have the organist play. A soloist was discouraged. Lyrics bring forth such strong emotions, and as we would be a small group in a small room, they cautioned us not to evoke an outpouring of tears. My sister and I walked quietly to our respective automobiles, having decided to speak later on in the day. We were both feeling the reality of the visit and needed to go off in our own corners.

In appreciation, I called Elizabeth when I got home "I will pass your teachings on to others," I said. When my cousin Mary telephoned to inform me of my Uncle Alfred's death, I told her, "Let me pass on to you a special gift I received at the time of my mother's death, Mary. Take a bubble bath."

The nurses and I formed a sisterhood. Sometimes I dropped back. I understood I could not be in charge of what I didn't understand. Rather than watching them, I went out of the room and sat in the upstairs den. As a child I had left the room habitually when my sister got her poison ivy shots. Instead of blocking my ears as I had done back then, I now prayed and meditated. When I prayed I asked for the strength and the courage to go on. During my times of meditation when my mind would unconsciously jump from thought to thought, I heard myself uttering words like those coming from a stranger: "Thank You, Lord, for solving my mystery. I no longer need to ask that agonizing question: which parent can survive the best without the other?"

Although I was particularly aware of my mother's frailty and vulnerability, I knew that I felt fortunate that I did not see her in pain. She may have hidden it from me; from her head to her fingertips she was stock stoic. I cannot remember a time when she was whiny or appeared to be feeling sorry for herself. It was disconcerting and upsetting for me to see her being taken care of. I did not want to watch. I felt it was humiliating for my mother. I had strong compassion for feeling weak, and I was determined to respect and love her for her strengths to the very end. I was also feeling, *My God, is it getting really close to the end?*

I didn't feel my father's physical deterioration in quite the same way I did my mother's. I saw myself in my mother, like I would see myself in any woman, because her body was more connected to mine. I struggled to keep myself intact. I had been told once that merging was a hazard for a woman; the daughter takes on her mother's death as her own, their bodies in a kind of resonance. I sometimes feared in the presence of my mother if I allowed myself to be pulled down into her low energy, I might lose myself. It took a concerted effort to take care of myself. I had always possessed an overactive imagination; now was a time to use it, to bring Mother a sense of cheerful connection with the things she loved in the past. In the playful determined way that I had always loved to communicate with her, I felt I was firing energy into her. In the process I was giving her the gift of my attention and my love. Whenever I succeeded in pleasing her, I felt I would later have no regrets. There was a way I was doing this song and dance for myself.

The bureau at the foot of my mother's bed became more comforting to me as her dying process progressed. I stood for hours at her bureau while she lay comatose in her bed. It comforted me to fondle her fine-textured hair net, like a baby plays with his mother's hair. "Mother, why did women with gray hair add blue to the final shampoo? Did it give the set added body? Or maybe it prevents the gray hairs from turning brittle." Like an adolescent child playing with her mother's makeup for the very first time. I was fascinated as I examined the array of items on her bureau tray. Mother, old-fashioned in many of her habits, wore lipstick primarily when "going out." I remember rolling the gold-colored tube around in my hand thinking how cold the shiny metal container felt in contrast to the warm springlike atmosphere of the bedroom. I squinted to read the worn seal on the bottom, MAUVE. I asked, "How is it your lipstick is shaped so differently from mine when our lips are shaped so alike? While mine is flat, yours has a peak on one side as steep as Mount Everest." As I raised the horizontal tube to my nose and inhaled deeply, I immediately felt myself falling into silent despair. The power of her familiar scent overwhelmed me with lively memories as I glanced over as her still body prepared itself for death. I think my mother knew how frantically I was summoning all my ingenuity to cheer her on because otherwise I would melt down with grief and helplessness. I'd read in books and seen on the screen how in other cultures they wailed and wept until the sorrow had been fully expressed from the whole body. On days when I was deep in the emotion of sorrow, I willed myself to wail, leaving empty pockets of space inside my soul for new life and revitalization to grow.

My consciousness was always divided. I could not allow myself to be drawn completely into Mother's dying. My father was downstairs. My thoughts would turn to him and his needs and my dread of displeasing him in any way. This judgmental, extraordinary man, grounded in the power of business ethics, like a warrior magician, could hit people between the eyes and leave them stunned. There he was downstairs and at any moment in his erratic behavior he might suddenly appear, in a fit of anger and tell me to leave and to take the nurses with me and that he would be caring for his wife himself. I was caught in a bind, wanting to be close to my dying mother to accompany her in her letting-go process and wanting to light candles, wanting to recite prayers aloud, wanting to step outdoors in the side yard and pick buttercups and look for four-leaf clovers, place them in small pottery jars around her room. Instead I had to keep myself very awake. There was a tyrant on the loose downstairs.

Because my mother was being taken away from me, I wanted to hoard her things. I had a compulsive urge to take half of Mother's hankies. The handkerchiefs were of old white linen, hand-rolled, with flowers beautifully appliqued with finely textured silver threads, and finished with French knots. They smelled like Mother. I feared the family would not see things the same way I did. I wanted all the hankies, but I was afraid that my sister would discover that I had taken more than my share. I knew this was childish. I remembered stealing my sister's colored pencils and colored elastic bands from a large red plaid pencil box my father had brought her back from New York. It was considered so special my mother had it stored in the attic until my sister was old enough to use it. Raised by an incredibly upright man and a woman who preached "share and share alike," I did not want to be the special daughter, taking advantage of my position. Although my sister had chosen to let me take on this position, I thought that perhaps others wondered how I had taken on this powerful role.

Like many other home-spun Yankee couples, my parents had always had a courteous relationship. During the final three days of my mother's life he did exactly want she asked him to do. Even with Alzheimer's disease he knew this was the end. My father sat downstairs in the living room silent and staring off into space, looking like a stranger lost on a mountain with unmarked trails. Puzzled and burdened by his lethargic behavior, I spoke to his nurse. "This may be his way of shutting down, a kind of depression," she said. This was the first time I had ever heard my father described as depressed. My father had always been the kind of man who fought to win. Yet once the end was inevitable he quietly let go. Businesspeople said of him, "He is not only a good loser; he has class." Just as I went out of my mother's room when the nurses were doing certain things, he didn't go into his wife's room while she was dying. As long as she was not asking for him he would not interfere. On a certain level you have to do dying alone. One doesn't marry for this reason. He was a man who knew how to protect himself, especially since 1958, when he suffered a heart attack. He was the same man who had left his car dealership so he did not have to see it burn. Standing in front of the showroom windows watching the fire engines round the bend, he had said to the salesman standing next to him, "No man should have to watch his life's work burn right before his own eyes. Call me at home when it's over." Later he was told, "Things don't look as bad as expected." Instead of fire engines, now it was nurses and more nurses coming to care of his wife.

Although my mother's bedroom was not lined with stained-glass windows like our church sanctuary, many days I was filled with a sense of holy acceptance when I walked into her room. Her condition no longer called for drama and pizzazz. She now required deep listening. For years I had been comfortable with silence and letting my body relax, even if my mind was drifting. In this simplicity I tried to take refuge. Having spent much of my life entertaining others, I yearned for that place inside myself where freedom ruled, where there was nowhere to go and nothing to do. I prayed for peace. When I felt the peace growing I let my tears flow, quietly. Not wanting to disturb the others downstairs, I controlled my sobs the same way one muffles a sneeze in church. I had never experienced the impact of sitting with someone who actually was dying. I grew to understand what it meant to open my heart endlessly. So close to the fundamental truth of impermanence, I began to consider my own passing. I wondered why death is sometimes slow. Is it because it is a preparation period for the next life? This thought gave me comfort and a certain warning.

I wanted to give Mother space and freedom for her dying time, recognizing her desire to be neat and efficient and get on with it. She had held on for her husband's sake. "Mother, I'm not so sure this is a good idea, your dying. Who will tell me to close the windows when it is about to rain? I need someone to tell me these things. You're good at that." That child part of me wanted my mother to go on forever. Sometimes it takes a child a long time to reach a place of wisdom, where she and her mother can communicate on the same level. In my adult years my mother and I set each other off like no one else could; we could belly-laugh about the silliest things. I'm grateful we had those later years together. I sat as close as I could without stealing from her any clear spring air coming in from the window. I remember, near the end, my stroking her arm while speaking aloud the inevitable: "Mother, I will miss you."

When the telephone rang, giving us the news, I remember consciously thinking of the birds singing outside our open bedroom window. Sybil's voice was clear and in control: "Janet, your mother died at four-thirty this morning. I was holding her hand." My first thought was to ask, "Why did someone not call me?" I thought of my father and his habit of being a light sleeper. There were necessary procedures to be carried out, preparation the nurses wanted to protect my father from seeing. At first these thoughts did not all come into focus for me. Why was Sybil talking about death certificate, signatures, the funeral parlor, and the body bag taking my mother away. What is a body bag? I had seen such things on the six o'clock news bringing young men home from foreign lands, but how did those canvas bags relate to my mother? I asked Gordon. Barbara and my preparations at the funeral parlor had not prepared me for this. I was in a dark forest where I had never been before. I was relieved when Sybil said she had phoned Barbara. I was not feeling up to making phone calls, even to my own children. I made a conscious decision to stay in bed and take it slowly, to begin the day with a bubble bath. I liked to think this early hour was part of God's larger plan. My father was home with people who not only cared about him but also understood how to respond to him. Leave it to my mother to die in a timely fashion!

Barbara and I had agreed to meet at my parents' house around nine o'clock. I was early. Our daughter Cindy was already there with Patrick, her two-year old son. My father was seated at the kitchen table, next to the window where my mother used to sit, having his coffee. He was a man who always liked having people around, and now they were his distraction. Because of his disease we did not speak of Mother, yet we were not denying her death to him, either. Sometimes it takes a child. When Cindy placed her son, Patrick on the floor he directly crawled over to where my father was sitting and hoisted himself up, using my father's leg for support, and laid his little head down on my father's knee and kept it there, as if to say, "Grampa Marble, I am so sorry." My father was so pleased and taken aback by this small child's gesture. He patted his head ever so gently.

I did not see Sybil that day. I suspect professional and experienced nurses plan it that way. They have their own letting go and grieving to do. Rhoda, the nurse, was now at the house and appeared to enjoy being nurse and maître d' to the grieving family. The nurses and our family went out of our way to be genuinely courteous to one another.

Yet I remembered what Elizabeth said about the danger of having our property stolen. Although this seemed hardly the case in our situation, one never knew. I came up with the idea of placing small white stickers haphazardly about the house, to indicate an inventory, of sorts, had been taken. Now that Mother had died and Daddy couldn't climb the flight of stairs anymore, the upstairs turned into a mausoleum. And that is what, I think, Barbara was feeling as we sat on my father's bed sorting out what remained of my mother's costume jewelry. "Please, Barbara, I know this is difficult and untimely, but we need closure upstairs; we still have Daddy to care for downstairs."

My sister mandated me to organize the funeral. I telephoned the same woman who so well catered my parents' mock seventieth anniversary party to let her know a funeral was in the making. I thought we could have the group assemble at my parents' house. I asked her to serve coffee, tea, nonalcoholic punch, and finger foods. I felt proud to deal with someone who had held my mother in such high regard.

I recalled the day when my mother told me to "be sure your father wears his newest gray suit 'that' day; I like the tie we bought to go with it."

"Red at a funeral?" I asked.

"They're wearing everything nowadays!" she said.

I had her already-cleaned grandmother-of-the-bride dress dry-cleaned once again, just in case it had gotten musty while hanging in her airtight heated attic. I purchased and rinsed out, for her, a new set of undergarments. I wanted these few things to be nice for her, like she had made things nice for me when I was a child.

I had written my mother's eulogy two years previously on the early morning of January 6, 1987, when she was in the hospital and the doctor said things were not looking good. *I'll write her a letter of love,* I thought. I had heard people say how putting feelings down on paper could be healing. I began by sketching, in outline form, her distinctive characteristics. Then I began to give snappy examples. As I wrote, I began to think of the people who would be invited to her funeral: employees of the dealership, old friends like Harry Harrison, and Eleanor, her hairdresser. By the time I finished I had covered three sheets of legal-sized paper, which I realized could become her eulogy. Now I rewrote it and asked the minister to read it. Mother would not have approved of our finalizing her burial arrangements within earshot of the nurse. Barbara and I made final arrangements privately standing outside our parents' driveway. As Gordon and I pulled into the florist shop to choose funeral floral pieces, I could see our three children waiting. I had telephoned them to invite them to join us in the selection of the flowers. When I saw on their faces the concern for me I realized I had invited them partly because I needed them close by. My Alzheimerish father was waiting for me.

Early the next morning Gordon went off to work and the children were home with their friends and families. There were times when I needed to be alone. I drove to Rye Beach to surround myself with pleasant memories of times with my parents there. Cruising along at a snail's pace, I drove down Sea Road, stopping now and again to take in the many changes over the years we had summered there. The old oak trees had grown taller and wider, forming an archway down to the foot of the street. I imagined my mother along with her brother and sister-in-law walking home from the Catholic church where they attended summer services each Sunday morning. I wondered now if my father had been invited and refused or if Mother had excluded him to have her family's attention for herself. I was reminded of the proverbial question, "How much attention does a woman get when there is a man around?" I stopped outside the house to reflect. When I was young the house had yellow awnings. Now they were gone, too. As I drove along the coastline I thought how ironic it was to have my parents live so near to the ocean when neither one of them swam or even waded. How different summers were before air-conditioning, when people, in the 1950s, moved to the beach simply to stay cool. I slipped my sandals off and strolled barefoot along the desolate beach. I thanked God for showing me His consistency through nature: for the unfailing salty tides, for the constant ebb and flow of each wave, and for the daily tempo brought about by sunrises and sunsets. The sky looked overcast with promise of clearing, an appropriate backdrop for my emotions. I wondered if my father, in his scrambled sense of loss, would be able to recall the day when he and Mother spoke of their final satisfaction with life.

I studied a formation of birds overhead, how when the lead bird got tired he rotated back into the formation and another bird close behind flew at the point position. I thought of Gordon and how willingly he had taken his turn, these past years, to do the hard tasks. I spotted a perfectly shaped sand dollar and bent down to pick it up. It was sandy beige with a hint of pink. As I traced my index finger along the center and around the edge, I thought about motherhood and its many cycles, about my children and their children and how it would be for me to be without a mother. For years now when I saw something pretty or was intrigued by something I heard, I held onto the thought, in order to share it with Mother; what would I do now, tell Daddy? I started to put the sand dollar into my pocket as a keepsake, then changed my mind. I'd rather hold onto this as a thought than take the chance of losing it, too.

I left the beach and stopped in at Jannett's, a popular shop for buying bathing suits. I wanted to ask the cute young clerk if she had a mother and did they shop together, but I didn't want to hear her answer. Thumbing through the racks, I found it soothing to play in this store as I had when I was a child. I found myself trying on big straw hats with large, colorful brims, hoping what I saw in the mirror would smile upon an otherwise sad face. On the ride home I stopped by to visit a woman who I knew would have a sympathetic, understanding ear, also a substitute matriarch in her family. We sipped lemonade and reminisced.

I was surprised when I arrived home to have flowers waiting for me at the door. I was inexperienced in funerals and the etiquette of having people come to the house pay respect to us as a family. As I look back, I didn't even serve them food. I dropped to an unfamiliar level caused by relief and grief together. When Gordon's sister and her husband dropped by I was quiet but cordial. I found I could rest now and let others find the right words. Feeling suddenly older, I sat on the couch thinking how beneficial it was for our children to have an opportunity to share with others stories about their grandmother.

When my friend and neighbor Cal came by the next morning with homemade hot blueberry muffins and with plans to return that evening at six o'clock with dinner, I saw this as a crowning and unique moment in my life. It made me feel proud in front of my children to have them see this act of friendship. When the Lynches called the next evening to take us out for a drive, "nowhere special and we'll keep it short," I was able to accept. By accepting people's kind gestures I was able to relinquish my dutiful feelings and enjoy being taken cared of.

At that time it seemed to me right not to rely upon the church for my strength. I was not ready to be out mingling with people; the church felt too social and threatening in my grieving time, although, I must admit, I did like it when one of the deacons stopped by that Sunday with the altar flowers and later that week when a member of the Thoughtful Circle dropped by with a single red rose to give her condolences in behalf of the group. Instead I privately wrote thank-you notes and walked the beach. Every morning for the next few weeks I was up at five o'clock on the dot. With the notes that I wrote to the nurses, I often included a little memento, such as one of my mother's hankies or favorite recipes. I made a copy of her banana bread recipe and gave the original to the nurse who had held her hand while she died. I chose to write to all of my father's professional colleagues and contacts, trying to use his words as well as I could, since he was incapable of doing so himself. I was still feeling driven to keep organized and in charge and accomplishing everything that I could. I handled my denial by passionately turning up my organizational flame, wanting to be best at what I am doing whenever I can be. It gave me a sense of pleasure and accomplishment.

This was the first funeral in our family of my generation, and I was acutely aware of my lack of experience. I decided to call the funeral director and ask if Mother could be "ready for a private showing" before the two o'clock funeral. I hoped this was not an unreasonable request. I wanted family members to feel free to have time alone with her and not to feel rushed.

One by one we scattered our visits throughout late morning and early afternoon, as we had on Mother's Day. Intentionally I was the last to arrive. The funeral director's wife, greeted me at the funeral home door. As she was a former tennis partner of mine, ordinarily we would have hugged. On this day she held back. I was grateful for her style and sensitivity. To feel her tightly wrapped arms round me would have been more than I could handle. Three days later I called and thanked her.

I was quite the businesswoman about what needed to be done, but I was devastated. I stood before Mother's coffin shooting last-minute questions like wobbly arrows in the air: *How do I care for Daddy without you around? Who else will I permit to stroke me as if I were a child? You are the person I have always relied on, and now you are gone. Where do I turn?* Gradually I pulled myself together. I could hear my mother's voice saying, "Janet, don't lay guilt trips on me. I'm already dead." I let myself speak of my love for her.

My mother had been a weather person. So when the sun appeared on the day of her funereal, after a weekend of rain, relatives commented on it back at the house. Family members chose to drive their own cars to the funeral parlor rather than be picked up by limousine. The children arrived together. Elizabeth, the nurse, drove my father. I wore a dress of which Mother would have approved. Both my daughters did the same. Mother had taught us to be fifteen minutes early to weddings and to funerals, but this time we went thirty minutes early. My father went to the men's room and then settled into a seat in the front row, close and in clear view of his wife. Elizabeth, wisely, let him be in charge of himself as much as possible. We did not want a scene. I watched Elizabeth lean over and heard her whisper in his ear, "Doesn't Al look peaceful, Ted?"

Most people had not seen my father since his official diagnosis of Alzheimer's disease, and I imagined how confusing it might be for them to meet him. I could see people begin to relax as they observed, from afar, his still-handsome physical appearance. He was dressed in his gray suit and red tie; shoes shined, his face not only had been freshly shaven but moisturized as well, and his long-standing white hair was thicker than that of both his sons-in-law. Close friends, employees, and extended family walked over to greet him before the service began;

the rest of us mingled with guests in the front vestibule. His Alzheimer's was working for him. Like an effective astringent it helped to take the sting away and allowed him to be sociable. He was cordial and witty; he rose to the occasion like a seasoned star.

I sacrificed my relationship to my own feelings in order to take care of him that day. I felt like a sentry keeping watch. I feared if he knew I was tense, it might trigger him off. I recall checking out if my shoulders and legs were relaxed. If I tightened up, confused and insecure, he would tighten up by expressing anger. I believed I had earned the right to be fully present at my own mother's funeral, but I was at the mercy of his irrational, tyrannical behavior. I got the idea to image myself split down the middle. I divided my attention as best I could between his needs and my own. I was able to wrap myself warmly in prayer and listen intently to the poems that were recited. I tried to find balance.

My parent's standards of courtesy prevailed throughout the funeral, I asked my two nephews to stand in front of their grandfather while the cover was closed on the open casket. Reverend Graichen suggested my father stay in the car with his window down and offered a prayer while standing next to him. Family members and friends were invited to surround the casket.

4

Be willing to have it so.
—William James, a nineteenth-century
philosopher-psychologist and spiritual pioneer

I preferred not to be depressed by my father's situation. I did not look for him to be the man he once had been; instead I looked for ways to enrich the man he had become. Rather than test his memory or correct his errors, I looked for creative ways to nourish him and our relationship. Every time I walked into his house I defined myself: "Hi, Daddy; it's Janet." Because in the old days he would have answered, "Good to see you," I added, "Aren't you glad I'm here? I am."

When I took myself to a health spa the week following Mother's funeral, I put up a good front most of the time. Fiery and decisive as usual, I searched actively for an environment where I could replenish sapped energy. I chose to attend the spa, where no one would know me. At the health spa I discovered that I liked people dressed all the same, in white terry-cloth robes. I knew I had to embrace my sorrow before I could let it go. I approached it in a businesslike way. Through focused imagination, I communicated with my pain. I talked into my tape recorder. Sauna and massage rituals helped. In humorous desperation I wanted to do something bizarre, as now would be a

Commonwealth of Massachusetts
CERTIFICATE OF MARRIAGE

I, Nancy F. Driscoll, hereby certify that it appears by the Record of Marriages in the said City, that a Marriage was solemnized between

........Albert D. Marble........ and ....Alice J. Heffernan........

on the ....7th........ day of ....February........ in the year 19.20.

GROOM		BRIDE	
Name	Albert D. Marble	Name	Alice J. Heffernan
Color		Color	
Age	21	Age	20
No. of Marriage	1st	No. of Marriage	1st
Residence	9 Victor st	Residence	7 Norfolk st
Occupation	Wood heels	Occupation	at home
Birthplace	Haverhill	Birthplace	Haverhill
Father's Name	Charles E Marble	Father's Name	Jean Heffernan
Mother's Name	Bertha Pressey	Mother's Name	Mary Heffernan
Place and Date of Marriage	Salem,N.H.		February 7, 1920
By Whom Married	John W. Clutter	Clergyman	Salem,N.H.

I, Nancy F. Driscoll, above named, depose and say that I hold the office of City Clerk of the City of Haverhill in the County of Essex and Commonwealth of Massachusetts; that the records of Births, Marriages and Deaths in said City, and of the former Town of Bradford, are in my custody and that the above is a true extract from the Records of Marriages in said City.

WITNESS my hand and the Seal of the said City, on the day and year first above written.

_____Nancy F Driscoll_____ CITY CLERK.

My parents' marriage certificate

good time, I thought, to have a drink and a cigarette. I made my smoke screen, balanced out by being at a health spa, and each afternoon I would drive two miles down the road to the local package store and purchase two, single-serving bottles of Fuzzy Navels. The crazy name was what first caught my eyes, and the exotic appeal of peach schnapps and orange juice. I threw in two packages of pocket-size Nabs. While the majority of ladies were firmly on power walks, I was in my room, stretched out on a boudoir lounge-chair. Each evening when I heard proud testimonies to the program, I sat graciously silent.

I called my father's house two out of three shifts a day; I would have called during the late-night shift as well, if I hadn't been afraid of waking someone or, in my

144

anxious caretaker's mode, thought of as "crazy." I made it very clear before I left home, when I telephoned to receive a report I didn't want to sit on the other end of the receiver and listen to my father awkwardly make his way to the phone. I didn't want him to become confused and angry because he was only hearing my voice. I wanted to avoid feeling intimidated and terrified on the other end of the line.

When I returned home I felt like a child on a seesaw sitting in anticipation, I was feeling tense and afraid. I had been caring for my mother, whose faculties were intact while her body was dying; now I was becoming primary caretaker of my father, who was mentally ill. Although I always looked for my sister's consent, I was his primary caretaker. My whole life was coming into a new balance.

My mother would have expected after she died that my father would go immediately into a nursing home. I thought to myself, *We need a new plan.* What worked for my parents as a couple would no longer apply. I remembered a conversation with Andrea, the nurse, while Mother was in the next room, lying on her deathbed.

Andrea said, "Janet, your parents have suffered from two very different sorts of illness. It will be unnecessary for you to care for your father in the same way you have cared for your mother."

As I listened intently I feared now that even she would encourage me to ignore him. Like a skunk, I felt the hair rising on the back of my neck. I knew Andrea was a member of the New Hampshire Hospice Program.

Puzzled, I asked, "Could you please give me an example?"

She responded. "Because your mother's mind has been clear and she has been able to understand the concept of time, you have strived to make your visits lengthy and pleasurable. Is that correct?"

"Yes," I softly said, feeling my defensiveness melting down.

She continued, "Your father's situation is just the opposite. I know he is able to read the numbers on his watch and state the correct time of day. He knows the difference between bedtime and mealtime. However, he does not know whether your visit has lasted five minutes or fifty minutes. This is why I suggest you keep your visits frequent but short. Twenty minutes should be ample."

As a family we were in mourning and feeling shattered. It seemed best for him to maintain his regular routine at home. There also was an ethical question. If our brave, clear-thinking mother was allowed the luxury of dying at home, should not her Alzheimer-afflicted provider be granted the same opportunity? Together we agreed to evaluate the situation again, at the end of one year. As I began hiring people and became the director of the drama, a crazily devoted daughter obsessed and compelled, I feared if I let myself down a little bit I could go all the way. I remembered my mother saying that about herself when she was ill. Instead I doubled, then tripled my efforts. When my children were young and going off to school, rather than saying, "Have a nice day," I used to say, "Make a nice day for yourself." I had read it once and thought, *What a great concept, and such a subtle, pleasant way to teach children to take responsibility for their lives.*

I did not want to be in touch with my sorrow. Just as a daughter can take on her mother's death as her own, I was determined not to take on the nothingness of Alzheimer's and go into that despair. Action was my camouflage. I chose to attend to him as a sacred being. I was less at the mercy of what came from his mouth or how he acted when I maintained an awareness of his spiritual presence. This made caring for him a spiritual deed. I was full of heartache some of the time and still bucked right up doing what needed to be done. I kept myself from being hopelessly sad by convincing myself that I was having the time of my life. Day in and day out I dressed myself up and put myself onstage. I was determined to make the situation work.

As I look back, I can see that as I was caring for my parents, the strengths that they had passed on were very much helping me to take care of them. One of these strengths was my father's extraordinary business acumen, his ability to take hold of a whole situation well into the future, with a six-month plan, a one-year plan, a five-year plan, etc. People often remarked on my ability: "It's amazing, Janet, how you grasp the situation so quickly and from so many angles." Looking back, I can see that perhaps I had developed this strength by studying my father. I took on many of his habits and attitudes: I had a deep feeling that I must not let the business fail. Very steady and very sturdy in my commitments, whatever I stepped into I had to make a "growing concern." Even now when I am angry at my husband, I ask to meet in the living room for an abjectly businesslike discussion. Business was the order of the day and not to be mixed with pleasure. "No business talk at the dinner table," you would hear my father say. In turn, I did not speak to the nurses regarding my father's health or behavior in front of him. If I was conversing with my father and a nurse wanted to speak with me, I would say, "I'm visiting with my father right now. We'll take care of business later, in the other room."

I learned from my mother to be territorial. Like many

women of her generation, she closed her eyes intentionally to her husband's work; she didn't want to know about it. I don't recall her ever asking how his day was at work; it wasn't her territory.

I had learned to identify texture when I accompanied my mother on shopping expeditions. Since she has passed on, I miss the way that she identified the quality of fabric with her quick, agile fingers. Together we had sought the best silk and linen; now I was looking for the best-quality support. Necessity is the mother of invention. Absorbed in a task that very few people understood, I felt vulnerable in my own hometown. I discovered that many people are reluctant to relate to people who are ill and dying. I felt the responsibility through every cell and pore of my body. I was tapping into my strengths with whatever ingenuity I could find. I drew on my power of visualization. If I was feeling duty-bound, alone, and in need of positive feedback, I practiced visualization, and I was good at it. Giving an emotion shape and dimension, richness of color, and tactile sense gave me an alternative perspective. Days I needed different forms of protection. When I was too tired to talk and wanted to be out of reach, I envisioned myself standing watch in a lighthouse where I could maintain a shining light for ships at sea.

Back then I was not an easy person to be around, nor was I an easy person to please. My friend Diane told me once, "You are a very hard person to do for." I can see now how it is difficult to be with a person who lives with such intensity. My adrenaline was at a high pitch. From the outside it looked as though I was much too busy to take in people's sympathy. Yet I wish someone had dropped off a simple gift like hand cream or an envelope of bubble bath, just a token, or a supportive message on my answering machine.

My father was a very demanding person to live with. He had very high standards. He had very strong ethical principles, and he was uncompromising. He was a man who lived, unchallenged, on top of his own world. With him there was no room to negotiate. My sister and I were not able to debate issues with him. Because of my parents' contrasting personalities, I never knew whether or not to speak up. As a child, I was torn between a mother who was telling me to keep still, bite your tongue, and a father who was asking me to explain myself. It was not unusual for him to challenge me with, "Janet, why do you say that?" I believe he was looking for his daughter's rationale, but sometimes it seemed he was just hounding me. Now as an adult I find myself stumbling over both styles of communication. Even when I know I have valuable information to offer, when I speak out I apologize for having something to say.

In her late sixties my mother fell down and broke her wrist, a bad break in a difficult spot to mend. Because she was incapacitated and alone a good part of the day, I came forth with an idea of which I thought my father would approve. When I walked into his office he welcomed me with a warm smile. I took my usual seat across from his desk. I was feeling relaxed and "cocky." My suggestion was to have Mrs. Philbrick, our cleaning woman, come to their house to help Mother prepare dinner. "She could even stay on to do the dishes," I said, "alleviating you from the job."

I knew immediately from the wild glare in his eyes that something was amiss. "Don't you ever come in here and tell me how to care for my wife or how to run my household."

Even today, although I am a strong woman who does not hesitate to say, "Don't talk to me like that," I can only say it to people outside our family and to my husband. I hesitated to approach my father ever again with any kind of suggestion. In retrospect, I can see it was his loss. I can also see now why it was so frightening for me to step forward in defense of my mother's daily care when she was gravely ill. As a devoted daughter struggling to earn her father's trust, I often shook like a child left out in the cold.

Ironically, I tried to create closeness with my father by emulating him. While my parents were ill and the house was in crisis, I increasingly learned to be the boss and in certain ways the tyrant also: "I'm in charge. My word is law and ethically sound because I think so. There is no room for negotiation because this is *it*. I'm the one who knows because if I don't know, this whole conglomerate is going down like the stock market crash of 1938." It would have been nice if I could have given myself a little more leeway; instead, every day was perfection at the "car dealership."

I seldom find myself without something to say, but the day Rhoda, the nurse, told me that my father was having sexual arousals due to his new medication, I found myself speechless. The situation took me completely by surprise—an unchaperoned nurse and a sexually wacky father. It was certainly an opportunity to go to the carwash. Then I thought, *How do I tell my sister*? He was not one of those fathers who went on sexual binges. For years at the dealership I saw how women were attracted to him, but he was a rock. The man wasn't even a flirt! It was no secret we had a particularly reserved and contained, strict and stoic proper family life. I remembered when, as I was a girl, the door closed to my parents' bedroom. I put my pillow over my head, when I heard them laughing, grabbed the other pillow, and slid down underneath my covers. Although I had gotten past the Victorian curtain over my parents' sexual lives, still, listening to the nurses was awkward and painful for me. Rhoda found the situation amusing and, in some bizarre way, complimentary. I listened to her with only half an ear. The other half of me was thinking, *What if this father of mine comes on to her and signs an affidavit turning his money over to a nurse, in hopes of luring her on?*

I put my good manners aside and quickly cut to the chase: "Call the doctor, *now* and have his medicine changed."

I was terrified that somehow during these sexual arousals, shifting around in his own memories he would confuse me for his wife. After all, I was in many ways representing her. I stayed away from him for the next couple of days. As I look back, I can see the devastating humor of the situation. I was not only in charge of the household but I also had become responsible for my father's sexual behavior, the last role I wanted to play.

I concentrated on being a strong-minded, independent woman. I thought to myself, *This is the next phase of my parent's development. It's a little bit difficult right now, but we have a job to do, and this, too, shall pass.* By no means was I to sit around and be depressed and helpless or to whine. I didn't become a bridge addict or hide myself in my children or say, "I'll have enough alcohol to knock myself silly at the end of the day." My father had been present in his business every day, and I was staunchly determined and conditioned to be conscious and present and effectual and to have an "in charge" attitude.

When I heard nurses whining about life in general, it enraged me. When others were depressed and disengaged I saw *red*. Yet there were times I felt sorry for myself. People put fear and doubts in my mind about whether things were progressing reasonably and made it even harder for me to feel right about what I was doing. When I caught myself and then bounced back, I wanted to say, "You damn fools, don't you get it? The situation itself is dark. When you surround a dark situation with dark energy, where do you suppose the light will come from?"

In order to *be* present in my father's house, I kept my eyes half-closed. Other people might try other escape routes, but this was my way. I had learned from my mother how not to look at what was really going on with my father. My mother's influence continued to impact me even after she died. Whatever was ugly, whatever was undignified, whatever did not reflect well upon her, she brushed over as lightly as she could. When he had been on one of his nightly rampages, the next morning she would minimize it. Rather than saying, "Janet, it's so painful for me to see my husband acting up this way; it just wrenches my heart. Sit here close to me, will you please?" she would say, "Your father was up to no good again last night." I knew she was protecting herself because she did not want to look at the disease head-on. What I did not realize was how I wore my mother's glasses. We spent more time on building our defenses than we did on expressing our pain. I compelled my own family to wear my glasses with me. Yet the nurses, in contrast, wanted to report everything to me. When they persisted with the grim details I was very angry, yet I kept it to myself. It was a terrible feeling for an adoring daughter to be embarrassed and ashamed of her father.

I had conflicting feelings because I was in a battle with the nurses and with myself. I was mourning my childhood. I was mourning the passing of my whole order of life that was slowly but surely out of my view, the tangible parts of it and the intangible. At first I didn't want anything changed, if possible. I wanted my mother still there, I wanted life to be going on as usual, and yet it was not going on as usual and I had to go along with the changes. While others were nostalgic and emotional I was digging my heels further to stay on-task. Stepping in without the buffer of Mother created a new set of feelings I had to deal with. I had worked so hard to maintain a high level of energy in the house. We had pretty much left the upstairs the way she kept it, but I refused to turn the downstairs into a museum to my mother's memory.

My mother had adopted during her final three years a certain relation to her husband. "He does not try hard enough and is too content to sit comfortably in his wing-back chair," she said. As his daughter now I was free to indulge the man who had always taken care of others. As his daughter I thought he needed to rest, to be cared for at last, with a healthy sort of indulgence. Changing details of my mother's housekeeping habits, I. felt at times strangely like my father's new wife; I was the one who knew him best, in his own house. For years he had been complaining about the scatter rug by the back door and the one going into the dining room. Why my mother had never discarded them was beyond me.

"Daddy, let's get rid of them. I'll put them down in the cellar rather than in the ash barrel, just in case—"

"Good," he replied. "I nearly kill myself every time I go to step over them."

I knew how important it was to make his house visitor-friendly. I thought to myself, *We need conversation pieces strategically placed throughout the living room.* "Daddy," I said, "let's get out the inscribed crystal bowl you received from Cadillac for fifty years of service as a dealer." I found it on the top shelf of the kitchen cabinet. He was pleased when I placed it smack in the center of the coffee table. When the sun shone from the bow window at the right angle, the bowl glistened, similar to the way his eyes glowed when people commented on his half-century accomplishment. Mother was no longer around to keep facts straight. I brought from the attic pictures of his youth and identified each person in writing at the bottom of the photo.

While my mother had paved the way for me to make changes, she also had passed the torch on to the nurses. Now her house never retired; it was in operation twenty-four hours a day. I noticed how the nurses kept the memory of my mother alive. One nurse would clean out the refrigerator while another, conscious of how Mother had liked to see her countertops cleared, would place the smaller appliances out of the way. Karen, one of the regular nurses, kept the ongoing grocery list on the mahogany table next to the telephone, "where Alice had it." Running our household twenty-four hours was a challenge to us all, even for those who came to visit. There were more days than I care to remember when I drove out the driveway wanting to wail. I would try to summon my mother's spirit and speak to my mother: "So *this* is what it was like for you, God bless you, and, God, please take care of me."

The grandchildren continued to take the initiative and visit their grandfather. After their grandmother died and her house was no longer filled with her joyful listening ear, Cindy, with her newborn and two-year-old son, dropped in regularly several times a week. My father got a "boot" when Patrick headed straight for the toys. Valerie visited on weekends when she was home from school once or twice a month. Jeffrey was at school in Chicago at the time and was home less often yet telephoned, often more than once a week, to ask, "How are things with Grampa?" I was delighted to watch the relationship of my children grow during those years. Yet I always said, "Just because you are home on college break or live nearby, don't feel it is imperative to go up and visit your grandfather. I know how hideous this is and how difficult it is to step close to this situation. Whatever you decide is acceptable to me."

I think my children gradually recognized I had mixed feelings about being primary caretaker. I rejoiced that they were taking good initiative for themselves, especially when my headaches were killing me or when I was worn out from the daily stress of watching, now, my father fail. From an early age they had learned to be managers, just as I had learned to manage my time, inspired by my self-made father and my very organized mother. I liked the fact that they spoke to one another about their visits. Jeffrey never wanted to go alone, so he'd set up a time with either or both of his sisters. Prior to the visit he would stop by the bakery and pick up enough cookies to fill the household cookie tin. I didn't tell him to. Valerie made sure she had her private time and spoke up to the nurses to assure her private time. Sometimes they asked me to give them some pointers on what worked for me and what I talked about during my visits. I would say very little. I knew by now that each in his or her way was a master companion and soul mate and I didn't need to put words in anyone's mouth or take away the special something that each would bring to the visit. I didn't have to go and improve on their relationship. I didn't fuss over them afterward, either. It was beautiful and reassuring to see there were good signs they might look out for Gordon and me—when the time came.

My father was now a single man and headmaster of his domain. I threw out all the "Mr. and Mrs. Albert D.

Marble" return address labels and ordered others, printed with his name only. I did not want people to hesitate sending him a greeting card because they were not certain if he still lived at home. At Christmas I wanted his living room filled with holiday cards. One crisp fall day I brought samples of Thanksgiving cards from which he selected one. I explained how his name would appear engraved just below the message. "The same way you and Mother handled your signatures on Christmas cards," I said reassuringly. My father had always been an appreciative man and had regularly given thanks to loyal friends, relatives, and employees who had been supportive to him throughout the years, sensing it instilled a renewed sense of community. I felt a special closeness to my mother's spirit as I copied names in her handwriting from her address book. For over a week, each morning, I sat across from my father at the kitchen table. With each card there was a story; with each story there was a special memory. We had created a special rhapsody of understanding with those Thanksgiving cards after my mother's death. When I kissed him good-bye, he would catch my eye, smile, pause, and then add, "You do good work." My father always appreciated effort. He respected it.

Whenever possible I gave him choices and encouraged him to think he was a codirector in this long-running show. Like when signing up for "perpetual greens keeping" of my mother's cemetery plot. I gathered all the information then, at the kitchen table, went over it with him in great detail. "What do you think?" I would ask.

Usually he answered, "Sounds good to me," or, "I'll go along with whatever you decide."

As he was a shrewd businessman and nobody's fool, ironically, it seemed to me he was not about to take the chance of making a wrong decision. I fed into his image of "proud father" by being boastful even though it made me feel silly and uncomfortable in front of the nurses. I recall the day I told him how I had planned to become a member of the board at the cemetery, in order to keep an eye on Mother's lot. "After all," I said, "I was the first female moderator of our church; I might as well be the first female on the board of directors at Linwood Cemetery." His eyes and broad grin told us how he loved hearing his daughter speak his language. I always left the best for last: "Daddy, you did such a good job in raising me. I could never have been so pushy if you hadn't taught me how."

He would laugh and reply, "I did do good work, didn't I."

I quickly put a positive slant on tragedy and treated it as a funny bounce of the ball. That is the same way I saw my father's Alzheimer's. He was still my father, a viable human being. I never saw him in pain or too weak to speak. We were regularly told his heart was strong and his blood pressure was in the range of normal. He did, however, have edema in his feet and his ankles and an ongoing battle with regularity. Time and time again I saw what life comes down to is a good belly laugh and a good bowel movement, both in the same day. A square fourteen-inch footstool was what he used to rest his feet on. He was capable of shifting around in his chair to make himself comfortable, but he was unable, on his own, to stand up. He needed someone to grasp both his hands and pull him up on the count of three. My father had magnificent long and thin fingers. I never remember seeing his knuckles puffy or disfigured with arthritis. He had wonderful command of his hands. When they were idle he kept them quietly folded in his lap. During the winter months he was in the habit of wearing gloves until his senses were dulled and he needed to use his fingertips as sensors. Handsome as my father was, his hands are the feature that stand out most in my memory. It was tricky getting him up from the chair at the kitchen table. That is why we substituted a dining room chair for it.

The family all knew he was not dying and what he really needed was to be well groomed, well fed, and well entertained. Unlike my mother, he did not experience mental anguish. He never gave the impression he might be longing for death to come more quickly. He spoke enthusiastically of living to be one hundred: "People don't give up on their cars; why would they give up on life?" I never saw the glimmer of hopelessness in his eyes, only in the eyes of those who stopped by to visit.

As nurses and family members we oftentimes asked ourselves, How much was dementia and how much was failing eyesight? The family wanted to have his eyes examined, but we were told by a physician there was no accurate way to take the examination. His eyes were where I first looked. They were my "cue" in this ever-changing drama. If his wonderful blue eyes looked clear and alert, I could relax a little. I could talk to him and he would nicely respond. I could make jokes and get him to laugh. But if his eyes looked narrow and slightly unfocused, with a yellowish film covering the pupil, then I had to be prepared to respond to another sort of mood, whatever it might be.

I soon learned that, as my father became more Alzheimerish, he needed and responded to touch more than the spoken word. The old rule of no kisses in case of germs was stricken, and a new rule emerged that I could kiss my father. He responded to the affection. My father was one who believed in the importance of holding an upright posture. He was no slouch! His neck muscles were beginning to weaken now, and I placed myself underneath the tilt of his head by sitting on my Aunt Beverly's embroidered footstool. Gradually I learned I could sit next to him and lay my hand on his knee to comfort him. There was something between us that made the placement of my hand on his knee all right. It was a gesture of tenderness as much as it was my attempt to help him focus on our conversation. He tried very hard to follow the conversation and to see with his hampered mind's eye the pictures I was sketching through my words. My parents had never been physically demonstrative, kissing or holding hands in public. I wish sometimes that I had gotten closer to them physically as a child. If they had been more of a feeling couple I would have thought to bring his pajama top up and put it close to her because of the scent. And I would have found a way to bring her perfume to him.

One day my father and I were seated alone in the living room talking. I paused for only a minute to catch my breath, but that was all the time he needed to lose his concentration. He started right in, "Tell those people to leave; I'm tired of them being here. They've been here all day and I'm tired of feeding them."

In order to validate what he saw, I asked, "What people, Daddy?"

"Those people down there at the end of the room, tell them to leave." I could tell by the tone of his voice that he was annoyed, not angry.

"Daddy, I have a problem. I would be very glad to ask those people to leave, but I don't see them—which doesn't mean that they're not there; it's just that I don't see them. Daddy, let me explain. I'm fifty-four and menopausal. Oftentimes when I'm boiling hot the rest of the world tells me it's cold. They call them hot flashes. Personally, I call them a nuisance. So call those people down there what-

ever you want, but I don't see them." I had him so confused that all he could do was shake his head in
wonderment.

I was wary of the nurses' comfort in our house. The
window shades became symbolic. They would position
them in a place I didn't want them, and I would correct it
every time I went in, only to return the next day and find
them back to where they were before. This infuriated me.
I wanted my wishes respected. If I had to battle I would.
Sometimes it felt like the fall of Rome in a way and that
the barbarians had invaded our domain. I wanted to keep
them under control so I could hold onto the old order as
long as possible. They probably had other things they
were concerned about at home and had energy left over to
do those, so that was good. It was exhausting. In the
course of a week there were six to eight different nurses. I
had to be addressed with due respect. These nurses had
different personalities and housekeeping habits, and
some were irritating to me. It was crucial to keep the
house accident-free in order to prevent liability suits. I
had a trained eye for this. As a child I had heard my father talk prevention control at the dealership, and Deb-
bie, the executive director of the Girls Club, was a real
stickler, too, in this area. In the winter we kept all walk-
ways shoveled. Not just for the convenience of nurses, but
in case of an emergency and an ambulance, with
stretcher, needed to move through. Nurses were to park
their cars out in the street and not in the driveway, even if
it was stormy. In case of fire or a power outage we wanted
their cars available and out in the open. I was training
two or three nurses, and those nurses were training the
others.

My real feelings were not circulating very freely. Instead, I was in the very same bind that I had been in when I was a child and my father said, "Be like me; face things head-on," and my mother said, "Be quiet and mind your own business; just do what you have to do." The drive of my father and the stoicism of my mother kept me rigidly centered, with fabulous headaches. I continuously longed and searched for a middle ground, a way in which to balance myself. After my mother died I was much more vulnerable than I'd ever been before. My anxiety put me into hypervigilance and hyperactivity. My nerves were on edge most of the time. My father was no longer reliable to me. Sometimes his mind shifted so many different ways it was like looking into a kaleidoscope. Dreading to meet him out of control, I called ahead of time to see if conditions were such that I would be able to step into the house. Expecting disaster, I thought it was my duty to stand on a storm watch with Gordon. I see now there were times when, lost in my high adrenaline, I did things I wouldn't ordinarily have done. One morning, at the grocery store, I saw a woman stumble and I said loudly, "Ouch." I had wrapped my brain around other people's feelings, even strangers.

> You gain strength, courage and confidence by every experience in which you really stop to look fear in the face. . . . You must do the thing you cannot do.
>
> —Eleanor Roosevelt

When I was centered I was able to experience joy. I knew from past experience that when I honored the difficult I lived most deeply and fully. People had told me before that I was a creative person, but now I was becoming aware of this surging creative direction of my thoughts, intentions, and will. I would catch inspiration. The universe came to help me. Some days I left the house feeling transcendent, both of us mysteriously lifted together! Yet as far as I know there is always a shadow for every strength that we have. Overloaded with fiery determination, sometimes I lost control over the swirling momentum. If I spiraled upward too far, the only way I could come down was to crash. Today I recognize the pattern of my drive and can sometimes stop myself in midflight with a gentle reminder.

I realized one day, back when I was in my midforties, that my life lacked contentment. Like chewing on a sponge, no matter how hard I bit down, life lacked substance. Designing my life had been my vocation; I habitually strove to create a well-balanced life, including in the equation what I believed to be its three essential components: nourishment for my mind, body, and spirit. When I was a student, my mind was continually being enriched. My work at the Girls Club energized me and insisted I be more creative. My volunteer work at the church reinforced my spirituality. When my mother thought I looked tired and was overdoing my outside activities, she'd joke, "Janet, when are you going to stay home and get in off the streets?" I had ignored her; now I began to consider her point. I realized I did not want to stay at home restless and jumpy, sitting on the edge of my chair.

I woke up one morning with a new resolve. "Fishing, I must take up fishing! It's what every creative, well-rounded menopausal woman should do in order to stop her mind from spinning in circles or flopping around like a fish out of water." Back then fishing was popular mostly with men and children. Youngsters, like my three-year-old grandson, George, had their own fishing poles, handcrafted sticks with a string for a line. Fly fishing for women had not yet become the rage.

Whenever I was about to embark on a new interest I would head to the library. The children's section with the benefit of visual aids and the good large print helped to get me launched. It was now midmorning and most children were in school. The librarian was chatty and eager to help, but I wanted to go among the books, to test the waters, to be alone. Seated in a child-size chair, I flipped through the pages of a book titled *The First Book of Fishing*. I was surprised at how commonplace the equipment looked to me: bobbers, hooks, fishing line, and bait. For years I had seen such items in the neighbor's garages, as well as my own. Yet I was now seeing the gear as if for the very first time.

I decided to fish from a pond rather than a lake. Logistically it made more sense. Round Pond was at the head of our street and in walking distance; I knew the area well. Gordon and I used to park there when we were high school sweethearts. Later our children skated and went ice-fishing there. I imagined myself fishing along the side of the pond, out of sight from passing cars yet in view of occupied houses. *You can't be too safe nowadays,* I thought. Fishing from the banks was also practical. Otherwise I would be tied down to a boat. Yet it occurred to me that I could use the canoe hanging up in our garage. How awkward would that be to carry? *I could always drag it,* I thought with growing enthusiasm, like a fish running off with the line. I caught myself. *Janet,* I scolded, *calm down.*

I pushed the thought, *What will I wear?* far back in my mind. Because I was learning something new I did not want my mind jumping all over the place. Where do I go for a rod? What is enough and what is too much money to pay? For years I had talked to the fish market owner about his early morning trips to the Boston Fish Pier. I wanted to learn. I wanted to be taught by someone close to the source. I drove twenty miles to the fishing tackle shop next to the ocean. Behind the counter, in front of what looked to be a row of javelin spears, stood a younger version of a well-seasoned fisherman.

I needed to better prepare for the unexpected. I did not like the feel I got from the smirking men at the fishing shack, but as usual my good manners prevailed. On the return route headed for K-Mart, I began to wonder, *Will I be measured for a fishing rod the same way I was fitted for skis?* This time I would not be influenced by color. I hoped they wouldn't ask me my weight, and if they did, I would lie.

I had heard once, "Fish bite better on cloudy days; on hot sunny days they stay at the bottom where it is cool!" The sun was two hours on the other side of noon, a little too warm for experienced fishermen but more than adequate for me, and I was going off to fish. Whether I caught a fish or not was incidental. I must have walked with strong, satisfied gait as I headed up the street to Round Pond. In one hand I carried my pole; in the other I continuously positioned my hat, a khaki-colored man's-style chapeau. For years it had been my all-purpose hat. Today I needed it to protect me from getting a hook stuck in my head. This was Gordon's suggestion; he also suggested I wear my sunglasses to shield my eyes. My five-pocket denim skirt served as my tackle box. I had a pair of pliers, several rags, and cotton-soft garden gloves in my rear skirt pockets, to cover myself and protect the fish from suffering. I was especially pleased not to be loaded down with extra gear. I had scrubbed off all the price labels, using polish remover on the more stubborn tags. Before leaving the house I ran through in my mind what I supposed to be good fishing etiquette. I planned to greet fel-

164

low fishermen with a nod of my head or a short side-to-side wave, rather than speak aloud and frighten their fish away. Anything beyond my first catch I would release.

As the breeze blew calmly across the water I could feel its stillness under my skin. I was moved by many hidden emotions. My soul felt alive; my body felt humble. What looked so natural from the edge of the pond had taken me forty-plus years to identify. An unexpected and overwhelming sense of insignificant reality set in. As my hook made contact with the water, circles appeared. I studied how they worked their way out from their center. In a broad sense what Mother had said was correct; I did need to come in, to take a deep breath, seek my quiet center, and push on.

When the children came home that afternoon they discovered an original print of a sunfish on the refrigerator door announcing my new direction.

I noticed that Rhoda had placed a dish of loose grapes on the kitchen table in my father's reach. She explained that his strength and his grip was deteriorating and his hands needed stimulation. Already when tired, he was being fed his nighttime meal. Gordon had suspected this on nights when he'd have dinner at the house and my father would not attempt to eat but told Gordon to eat. By July 19 my father showed visible signs of Parkinson's. His hands shook and he shuffled, even more so, when he walked. I could not ignore it, I tried first to look at his new development from a professional point of view. I thought, *I'll buy some clay.* Then I thought, *No, it's too stiff. I'll buy Play-Doh instead. He'll find the iridescent colors uplifting and it will attract the grandchildren while the grown-ups visit with him.* There was a fine line between offering him

165

articles with therapeutic benefits and entertaining him the same way one would a child. We were not lowering his standards to child's play because he had Alzheimer's; rather, we were addressing his small motor movements, hoping this would have a refining and soothing effect. To sculpt Play-Doh at the kitchen table with my father was in many ways a labor of love. I had "the gift of gab," but I never had felt creative with my hands. The furthest I went was to knit Argyle socks for Gordon when I was in college and to take sewing lessons later when I was married. At church Christmas fairs I provided refreshments and supplies while the others did crafts. I remembered sitting in my grandmother's parlor watching her sew rugs. By hand she would stitch long strips of fabric together, then coil them into a circular pattern. I made "rugs" by rolling the Play-Doh between both my hands slowly and methodically, in order for my father to receive benefit from the smooth rhythmic motion. Then I would mold it into circular patterns. By mixing the colors I got a tweed effect. All of this we did while seated at the kitchen table. On days when I was less inspired, I made pizzas with him.

One evening Gordon came home with a set of twelve artistically designed miniature antique cars. The tires were very small, but they moved. As my father was a longtime automobile dealer, these cars awoke memories for him. Because they were solid he could move them around and grip them better than he could the soft Play Doh; I think the cold temperature of the metal gave more feeling to his fingertips. I added a few more popular models, with children he had observed and taught. Now, with visiting children, he would pretend to make a highway around the dish of grapes and the salt and pepper shaker.

I had read once that "soul food" is our passport to the

past. My father had not had the pleasure of smelling or tasting the flavor of charcoal-broiled food since we had spent summers at the beach and he cooked on the outdoor grill. The thought clicked in my mind to purchase a portable cast-iron hibachi. For safety the hibachi was to be kept on the porch. I decided that on days when I questioned a particular nurse's familiarity with grills, I would simply announce, "Cooking outside is off-limits today." I had the store clerk take the hibachi out of its carton. There was no need to confuse and distract my father with needless wrapping. I thought it would be amusing to stroll into the house with it. I was always looking for the drama in any situation.

One clear autumn day in October I found a high-tech apple peeler and slicer at Haverhill's newly opened gourmet shop. It was sturdy and made of enamel cast steel, with a stainless-steel shaft and prong. It had a suction base for gripping the counter, not unlike my mother's meat grinder that she retrieved from the cellar whenever she was about to make hash. While at the cash register paying Lillian, coowner of the store, I explained how by turning the handle my father's shoulder and hand dexterity might improve. "You may want to tell other customers who are in similar circumstances," I added. "Or maybe it would be good public relation strategy to donate a few to nursing homes or housing units for senior citizens." I was definitely "out of my tree." I couldn't wait to show Rhoda and my father: "Imagine the kind of feedback he'd get by handing out his own homemade candied apples for trick or treat on Halloween. He'd only need sixty or so. Maybe we would all go and pick apples together?"

The idea fell flat. He had told people for years, and was still telling us, "I can only do one thing at a time." He knew he couldn't manage both the turning the handle while keeping a watchful eye on the unraveling skin. He knew enough not to even try. Yet he benefited by watching Rhoda make pies. He could sit for two hours comfortably, like a child, while she kneaded and rolled out her dough and fit it into a plate. I knew that this was good for him because I'd watch his shoulders drop and I could see his face relax. As we strategized to make his life as pleasant as possible, cooking activities became so successful that during the holidays we encouraged the nurses to cook even more, by cooking for themselves. At Thanksgiving and Christmas I filled my mother's kitchen shelves with ingredients for fresh cranberry sauce and fillings for pumpkin, apple, and mince pies. I loved to please my father's palate. One day I heard him say, "When I was a child my mother cooked me Swiss chard." I thought to myself, *I didn't know that.* The next day, when I went up to visit, I brought a large brown paper bag full of Swiss chard and placed it on the kitchen counter. Rhoda, the nurse, steamed it and served it for lunch. After he complimented her on a "good-looking lunch," he then turned and asked, "Where's the vinegar?"

I was always searching for new activities to stimulate my father. I felt a passionate need to keep him from drifting into nothingness. My sister oftentimes said to me how she was concerned that the nurses would become bored and quit. It was then I thought to find creative activities that made sense to me and that would incorporate both my father's needs and the nurses' as well. One day it occurred to me to fill the house with smells that would invoke the past. Some people lose their sense of smell when they get old; my father lost his sense of self, but his other senses appeared intact. Why not have the nurses go ahead and do some family cooking here? They could sup-

168

ply their own groceries and containers; we had all Mother's unused seasonings to provide. At first the nurses were hesitant; they were not sure they could do it right. Ethically and professionally it went against their grain, but once they saw the benefit to my father, it was fine. Some nurses even brought their own dinner vegetables and let him watch while they cut the vegetables up ahead of time.

In my father's world, which was frequently out of kilter, the kitchen was as mystical as a monastery. He had always had an appreciation for good food, but now with Alzheimer's it was burgeoning. Rhoda, the seven-to-three nurse, who was just this side of middle age, cultivated many of the kitchen activities. While stirring cookie batter in his presence she would stir a memory or two. The regular and rhythmic motion would soothe his nerves and helped calm his breathing. During the hours when the scent of cooking was not filling the kitchen she would simmer a potpourri of spices on the stove for comfort. I was acutely aware that the life of a nurse is circumscribed by sickness and death and that our relationship would end abruptly someday. I didn't like that, yet I understood. It was consoling and comforting for me to be able to be delightfully creative. When I put whole vanilla beans into the rum bottles and labeled them "Pure Vanilla Extract," I knew that the nurses would remember how much I appreciated them two years from now, even though I would never see them again. That felt important to me. Little creative deeds helped me to focus my attention on positive action, which helped to keep my mind off my deeper feelings, my worries and anxieties. I was looking around the Alzheimer's and behind it but not at it. This was the great gift of being trained in denial. It was through the senses that I was connecting my life to his life. I wanted that life connection wherever I could find it, and I had the ability to stay focused and forget everything else.

I watched others develop their unique connections with my father during the months that followed. Every other week Gordon would go up to the house and have dinner with my father, alone. Gordon referred to it as "Men's Night." He would bring along new-car brochures with updated color charts and old photos of awards that my father had received from General Motors, sense memory-based items.

In February 1990 Gordon told me he had ordered, through the Kiplinger Letter a birthday card from the president of the United States to be sent to my father in recognition of his ninetieth birthday. I was surprised to hear that such a courtesy was available but not the least bit surprised that Gordon had arranged it. On June 22, the day before my father's birthday, I got an excited telephone call from Rhoda, the nurse. "You've got to come up here and see for yourself. Your father has received a personalized card from George and Barbara Bush and he is thrilled out of his mind. He is so proud he doesn't want to let it go. He even held onto it while eating his brownie."

We didn't have individual shifts on the weekends; instead Elizabeth stayed both Saturday and Sunday, until five o'clock. Saturday for my father was like a day at a luxury spa. Elizabeth would give him a facial by applying steam towels, cream, and gentle massage; he showed signs of psoriasis and she wanted to keep ahead of it. She would clip his toenails and give him a manicure. In the afternoon she would take him to her beauty parlor, where he got his haircut. "I used to pray with him that we'd have a safe drive," she said. Sometimes they would go to mass. One Sunday night, she told me that when he noticed people walking down the aisle carrying candles, he turned to her and said, "Do you think that would help me?" He was the kind of man who wasn't going to miss out on anything. Other times, Elizabeth reported, he would come out saying, "Didn't that man in front of me have a nice haircut." And then go on about how it was parted right and how he must have a good barber.

Karen and other nurses would look to my father for advice on their car and house insurance policies. In some ways he was still able to hold onto his good salesman and fatherly image, and this amazed me.

Although my father seldom listened to music, he had a wonderful ear for words. He gave his full attention to whoever was speaking to him, even when he was feeling cantankerous. He had always been considered a good conversationalist, but now I wanted to find a way to communicate where I could be in charge. I spoke up to his intelligence and not down to the Alzheimer's. In the same way he never spoke down to his grandchildren but rather raised them up. I strived for the right balance of humor and quality in our daily conversations. Because my father's memory was impaired I felt the pressure of making myself understood the first time. I suppose I could have said to myself, "What difference does it make what I say? He'll never remember it," but that was not my style then and it's still not my style. I was raised to meet the challenge and not to look for the easier path.

I had learned from attending storytelling workshops that "pure storytelling is when the storyteller had absolute faith in the power of the story." I especially spoke to him of memories. I was drawn often to speak of my grandmother, his mother. By pulling forth the richness of the past I was viewing my childhood in fresh new ways, which often surprised and delighted me. I never knew what would come forth next. I was as much intrigued as my father with myself and the process. On days when our combined energies were strong it was like we were in the middle of a dance and I was leading. There were days when I left my father thinking suffering is grace. Sometimes I found that I was relating to my father on another plane of consciousness, one that had no time or boundaries. In a context larger than life itself, it was like sitting in the quiet mystery of the universe, without judgment.

When I stumbled onto an attitude, an activity that worked, I stuck with it. Creating visual images had a powerful effect on my father in much the same way as visualization had on me. I led with special images from earlier years, such as my grandmother's cellar, its dirt floor and the damp smell of the stone walls. Rather than search for words to describe the sense of smell I simply raised my hand under my nose and gently sniffed. Some days I noticed his eyes following my gestures with relaxed intensity. I saw the positive results by the deep focus of his eyes; he looked like a man in deep thought. When I questioned whether or not my images were getting through, I ignored my doubts. As a child I was oftentimes told, "Janet, slow down and take a breath. Don't talk so fast. What's your hurry?" One day I discovered it was easier for him to follow my thoughts if I spoke slower than normal and with distinct clarity. Now and again when I sensed my energy was too high I pulled myself in and mirrored him instead. I incorporated well-defined hand gestures in order to focus his attention even further. When speaking of any kind of touch, I would lift my right hand to eye level and run my thumb slowly and rhythmically back and forth along the tips of my four fingers, yet not so long that it would mesmerize him into sleep. By doing this I was able to hold his attention and the attention of

172

other Alzheimer patients later when I ran a reminiscence program at an Alzheimer unit. Strong body language allowed me the use of fewer words.

One day I recognized the need to bring more people into the house to visit my father. At first I didn't know what to do. It was then that Gordon suggested we invite Charlie, my father's longtime friend, for lunch. Because he was diagnosed as legally blind and lived forty miles south of Haverhill, Gordon offered transportation. He would telephone him on Monday and ask, "Charlie, are you up for a visit?"

"You bet." You could hear the joy in Charlie's voice. With his raw wisdom Charlie had not only been my father's friend of fifty years; he also had been in the automobile business until his eyesight failed him. He had a unique sense of humor and a story for every teaching.

Gordon and I made sure that Charlie did not overstay his welcome and would come again. I let my father and Charlie visit alone, sensing a three-way conversation might be too much for us all. Beforehand I'd bring out old photographs of times when Charlie and his wife with my parents had traveled together. I placed a high-intensity magnifying glass next to Charlie's usual chair. Karen served lunch in the dining room rather than at the kitchen table. The following day, when Gordon called to thank Charlie for coming, it pleased us to know that he had not only been helpful to my father but had received some pleasure, too.

Willis, age eleven, also visited my father on a monthly basis. Willis's first visits were motivated through a Grandparenting network program at our church. He sat on the footstool at my father's feet and talked cars while his mother sat in a chair to one side.

Young and inquisitive, Willis was eager to hear all aspects of the automobile business. My father liked to talk about the days he was a mechanic and his dealership so small that he had to back cars in when working on the rear ends. Rhoda, the nurse, would serve homemade chocolate chip cookies and milk and the following day would write Willis a note thanking him for the visit and sign it from my father. One Saturday, Gordon took Willis down to the dealership and gave him a tour. He rode the dollies, examined the tool boxes, and experimented with the car wash. When my father died Willis wrote me a note of sorrow. Later we went out alone for dinner and shared memories and key chains and tokens of my father.

It would have been excruciating for me to be fired by my father. My father could be very forgiving, yet I didn't want to be caught short in his eyes. I had a horror that if he should regain his senses and start to interrogate me I somehow would not be acceptable in his eyes. I feared losing his love and esteem. His judgment came down so hard and absolute. When he was angry my dread and fear knocked my sorrow out into oblivion. I learned never to try to reason with him once his anger kicked in. Instead, I learned how and why to take flight. I had two different methods of leaving: when I saw the Alzheimer look in his eyes, I would appeal to his fatherly instincts with, "Daddy, I have to leave now. I have a dentist appointment in twenty minutes," or simply turn on my heels and walk away. I cooled myself down by taking myself through a car wash, sometimes as often as three times a week. The car wash attendant, like a ski lift attendant, was always there to put me on track. The water coming from all directions, I would release a big sigh, place my hands in my lap, and close my eyes. As I listened with a soft ear to the steady surge of water swishing against my car I imagined it running down my arms and out my fingertips. The sound of soapy water on the windshield reminded me of summer camp and stormy nights when I fell asleep to the smell of pine needles and the sound of rain landing on our cabin's metal roof. The floppy brushes and the cool rinse soothed my stress, washing it away. When I moved into the sunlight from behind the chamois curtain, today the show was over, I had come our sparkling fresh, ready to go home.

Sometimes my father's rage caused tangled feelings in my gut and dryness in my mouth. I didn't know whether my fear was causing me to panic or my panic was causing my fear. My terror would escalate through the crown of my head. The whirling of intensity made me afraid that I might be going "bonkers." I was mature and educated enough to know I did not have to continue this role forever. Trained to live a life of action and responsibility, I had a gift of transforming feelings into positive action. I persevered even though I was thinking, *How could this spoiled and overindulged man be so unreasonable?* Never hollering back, never impatient, I would stand rigid while my jaw was set to "do battle." I enunciated my words and fought to sound reasonable. My father had a keen eye for my expressions as well as for my emotions. He knew when I was up or down or worried, and I was hoping that he'd pick up on my reasonable tone, yet my controlled demeanor did not always calm his.

My child self was terrified to see my father, at the peak of his rage, when he was on the verge of being physically out of control. I was afraid that he might come at me and hurt me. I knew he had raised his hand to my mother during one of his bouts, maybe more than once, and to others also. I did not want to face that my perfect gentleman of a father could hurt somebody. As his daughter, I felt safer relating to his positive characteristics, idealizing him, rather than seeing his cruelty, selfishness, close-minded, judgmental habits and attitude and now his sudden outbursts of anger. If I didn't see those ugly characteristics in him, then I also didn't have to look at some of the same ones in myself.

On those days when I was feeling terrified, helpless, and hopeless and the car wash was not cooling me down, I brought myself to a Catholic church, because I knew it was always open. I did have my own pastor and my Sunday services were a support, but I needed church on weekdays also and alone, without the stress and strain of looks, questions, comments to add to my sense of exhaustion. I knew by the number of cars in the parking lot when I could be alone. Then I headed straight for the front pew. I would always genuflect, then bless myself. Gordon told me years back, when he was a pallbearer for a friend, how the priest in charge said to the non-Catholics, "When in Rome do what the Romans do." However, I didn't go up to the rail. I held my head high and made desperate eye contact with each of the three statues. I found I could light candles. I wondered whether if I left more dollars God would notice me more.

On those dark nights when Sundown Syndrome set in and there was no light I could only imagine what my mother had thought. Perhaps my father had not been a safe individual for her to relate to for many years, when he was domineering, not leaving her a squish of space. I accept now more of the inner truth of my parents' emotional lives, compassionately and realistically. I see the consequences on me and my sister. I see that they were real people who had their own struggles and their own shut-down places they could not get open again. Like my mother I, too, was now saying, "This I will deal with, but beyond that *no.*" I turned over the worst of the care to the nurses and to Gordon. I knew that had I exposed myself to my father's incontinence, violence, and shouting I could not have walked into his house each day all smiles. Because of the way I structured my life I was able to avoid the worst of Alzheimer's. I needed to be able to deny this messiness in order to feel safe enough to return each day and be "up." Nevertheless, I knew what the worst was; I was avoiding it by choice.

Even though I was not dwelling on the losses, I clearly was suffering. I had lost my childhood home; it now smelled like urine from the bedclothes they carried to the washing machine. In the beginning the odor was there now and again, but near the end it became a continual irritant to me. It was in the laundry, in the air, all through the house. I put vinegar dishes behind the draperies. I'd heard that was very good at absorbing odors, but it didn't help much. The smell of urine lingered on my clothing like perfume lingers on a shirt collar. It was further disturbing because I was not accustomed to relating to my father's lower anatomy.

His whole image, now, had broken down. One of the handsomest, best-groomed men in town had unkept hair and didn't even know it. I was seeing the pillar of reliability, predictable as the clock, losing control over all of his faculties and his physical body. In the midst of fooling myself, I created an environment where I was a stranger in my community. I lost my security when I went out; people were curious about the very things I was busy trying not to relate to. I was the daughter of a man with Alzheimer's, which to some was "the daughter of a dying idiot." I'm sure I cut many people cold when they extended me sympathy. I feared their softheartedness would pull down my energy. Like a child with a blanket. Rather than sit with my sorrow, I swung into action to try to get the very best for him: colorful striped shirts with button-down collars, washable khaki pants, and belts made from fabric rather than leather. I made sure he was dressed more like a college student than a feeble old man. I wanted people to see him at his best.

My father had an insatiable need to learn. In his conversations he earnestly drew people out. He always focused on them, their needs, and their concerns. From my mother, however, he had learned lightness and laughter, and this began to shine more and more freely. I was fascinated by his change of personality. I kept studying it. Sometimes I thought it was his Alzheimer's, and other times I thought it was the result of his retirement.

It was two years and two weeks to the day after the death of my mother when the family put all the pieces together and knew it was time to admit my father into a nursing home. He was getting weaker and more difficult for one person to handle. Yet it was my intention to make his life work and to attend to that with every fiber, every cell. I relied a lot on Elizabeth and her gut reaction to situations. An administrator at the Northeast Rehabilitation Center, it was her job to be an advocate for patients; she was all business and clearly had no hidden agenda. Together with my sister we decided to move him during the summer months; some of the family were concerned with his deteriorating mobility and fearful of a liability issue should he become even more violent.

The entire family was experiencing all the emotions that go along with extraordinary moments: resistance, relief, worry, and the usual fear of the unexpected, which wove its way precariously throughout his Alzheimer days. I felt particular compassion for my sister. I saw how the fear of the unknown immobilized her. Just the mention of the Alzheimer unit terrified her, making her unhinged and restless. I referred to it as "the Unit." I felt immense gratitude to the Glynn Nursing Home for recently setting up the Alzheimer unit. I saw that people were really being taken care of there, with some real creativity as well. It was well organized, with no clutter. The floors were shining; the walls were white; there was a sun parlor and also an outdoor patio where patients in nice weather sat at round tables with attractive umbrellas surrounded by nicely trimmed shrubs and colorful flowers. I was assured that there were no visiting restrictions and that I would be welcomed and encouraged to keep my regular visiting pattern.

Because we had already registered my father at the Glynn Alzheimer Unit, all that was left to do was make the telephone call. Barbara felt we should keep his house intact for one year, and I agreed, just in case. . . . The worst that could happen was that he wouldn't like the Unit and would insist on coming home. I also was concerned that after one or two days of cantankerous behavior he might be asked to leave.

I had already nurtured a relationship with the director of admittance, so when I telephoned Connie to say, "It's time," I was not speaking to a stranger. This felt important. When my voice cracked and the tears rolled down my cheeks, I just let them come. In three weeks, August 8, 1991, he was to arrive in the morning, at ten o'clock. As if he were a child at summer camp, we were requested to drop him off, quickly leave, and not return again for three days. This plan was to aid in his transition.

During this time of transition, I was like the mother

179

of a sick child. I had sent children off to camp and to school; Gordon and I went on a clothes-shopping spree for my father with a list so complete you'd think we were sending him off in search of a second wife. Once the middle-aged clerk learned we were there to purchase a new wardrobe for his upcoming move into an Alzheimer's nursing home, she joined in with real enthusiasm. Taking his reputation for being a well-dressed man one step further, we were looking for him to be noticed, not to enhance his ego but to stimulate friendly conversation. Knowing that people are fearful and hesitant to speak to an Alzheimer patient, by dressing him to the "nines" we would give people a place to begin: "Ted, don't you look nice today." I obsessed about his clothes. He had always worn solid white and blue crisp 100 percent all cotton shirts. Now we were selecting fresh and bright-colored stripes and coordinated those with a familiar loose-fitting cardigan golf sweater. Earlier on we had switched from worsted wool to washable wool, wrinkle-free trousers. These we had professionally laundered where the detergent was strong. On some level I must have known I was being wasteful buying him new underwear, but, as queen of denial, I just let it go. I bought two nightshirts with the intention of having them snipped up the back with velcro inserts, my own version of "the johnny." Later I found them in his bureau unfolded, never having been worn. He sat with his feet stretched in front of him, therefore I wanted him to be familiar with what he saw. I had to search in many stores until I found men's long black support stockings for his swollen ankles. Controlling and obsessive as I was, nevertheless I didn't insist he wear a necktie and be mistaken for the chairman of the board.

The next afternoon I dressed carefully to make a good

impression, put on my best scarf, and went off to meet the charge nurse of the unit. I asked Elizabeth, who was professional and precise and spoke the health care language, to accompany me. My nervous energy was power-packed with what I had been doing with my father for such a long time, and I was continuing in that mode. Focusing on making his life good helped me to escape from the grief of relocating him. The sight of the nursing home located directly across from the hospital gave me a fresh sense of reassurance. The furniture was less ornate than that in other nursing homes I had visited, the standard leather-like wingback chairs, a couch with no throw pillows, and two sturdy-looking mahogany end tables. Only the entrance portion of the lobby was carpeted. In Connie's office there lay a folder with my father's name printed across the top. Included in it were forms of various colors: the system was soundly in place! I eased back in my chair, my hands folded in repose, a habit I had learned from my father. I was trying very hard to be genuinely friendly.

We learned that the nurse-to-patient ratio was four to one. My sister and I had agreed that we would ease my father's transition by sending private nurses for three shifts a week. Through hard work he had earned and saved an unusual amount of money available to have him in the Alzheimer unit; one of only two patients who fully paid the bill was what I was told. We didn't want him to feel that all of sudden he was alone. I knew this was unusual for a private unit, but I also knew that my father's behavior could be extreme and that we were on a storm watch! The family was willing to cooperate on all levels, I had no idea convincing her would be that easy. I didn't have to persuade her. The director simply nodded her head in approval. I prayed *Thank You, Lord; thank You.* I asked the same questions any caring parent asks when sending her only child off to camp or school: "Do you have a standard clothes list? Who supplies the laundry bag? Do you only allow electric razors? By the way, what do we get for two hundred dollars a day?"

When it came to my father I could readily find anything to fuss and craze over. I was crushed to learn I wouldn't get to sew labels into my father's clothes the same way Mother did when she packed my sister and me off to camp. Instead we were to use laundry pencils, black. Indelible markers belonged on laundry bags, I thought, and not scripted across my father's freshly pressed shirts, yet if cloth labels got torn and lost in the laundry, the marker would do.

When it was Elizabeth's turn to speak, she didn't ask. She informed: "Ted is very clean. He will ask to wash his hands before and after each meal. We want his shirt covered when he eats. We care about his diet. For years he knew what was good for him and would eat the right amount. He still enjoys food yet forgets when he has eaten and asks to eat often. We use fresh fruit for a snack and as finger food; this helps to keep the circulation in arms moving and his fingers agile. Every morning he has a banana. We give him one teaspoon of Metamucil and four ounces of prune juice twice a day morning and night. We try to have him drink four to six glasses of water a day. I have a list of medications here you might want to go over. Do you wish us to bring his walker, commode, and wheelchair along with him?" As Elizabeth was speaking, Connie was writing everything down. Sometimes she would write the same thing twice, but on different forms. Whatever she was doing, I was continually reassured they would be proficient at meeting his needs.

I was relieved to learn that my father, diagnosed with advanced Alzheimer's would be put with a higher-functioning group for meals. Connie explained that he and ten others would be taken by elevator to their own private dining room. There he would be seated at one of the two round tables with a floral centerpiece, covered with white linen. They would be served traditional foods and eat from china. I remembered suddenly that my father's dental bridge had been slipping. We would need either to get it fixed or have it replaced. Gordon would find a local dentist.

The elevator appeared deeper than any I had ever seen. Its steel walls were soft beige and not padded. The lighting was more than sufficient; I was grateful, as one who resists gloom and doom on all levels. Along three of the walls was a chrome railing. There were many days, over the next several years, filled with crippling emotion after leaving my father, I felt the rail was all I had to hold onto until the touch of cold metal would wake me up to reality and I would remember my supportive family at home. The moment the elevator door opened the smell of urine assaulted the senses. The taste of fear began to form in the back of my throat. As Elizabeth stood on one side and Connie on the other I wondered if the odor of mashed carrots, potatoes, and meat nauseated them, too. In a calm manner I pushed my imaginary "pause button," raised my eyes to the ceiling, and begged, *Please, Lord.*

The nurses' station was located twenty feet from the elevator smack in the middle of the unit. In one sweep the nurses could view everything: both corridors, the entrance to each bedroom, the sun parlor where the more highly functioning people sat, and the activities room where, I later learned, the less coherent people were placed. It was touching to watch Connie and the nurses respectfully interact with the patients. Elizabeth's approach to the patients intrigued me. She would look them straight in the eye and say something like, "My, don't you look pretty in red." *Janet,* I said to myself, *you can either stand on the sidelines and wring your hands or do something.* Taking the smallest of baby steps and using great caution, I walked over to a lady I later knew as Hariette and said, "I like your aqua jogging suit. Aqua was my favorite color when I was a child." She smiled back. . . . I moved on.

Connie suggested to arrange my father's room at the Alzheimer's unit the day before his arrival. This distracted me from the magnitude of my loss. I knew I would eventually make a contribution in there. I was sensitive about my family's status and my father being a highly successful Cadillac car dealer. People often assume Cadillacs generate more profit than a less costly car, which is not so, yet I knew that private duty nurses on the scene would only add to this impression. I didn't want any resentment to be taken out on my father. It was important to me people meet him and me with respect, but not because of money. I didn't want anyone to think I was too privileged to be likeable or too spoiled not to know how to work. I carried in furniture and arranged the room alone; I wanted them to see I could work although I was sad.

People had heard of my maiden name, even if they had not bought a car from Marble Motors. The company, which had been in business for seventy-odd years, was in a busy square, adjacent to the downtown area. I introduced myself as Janet, Ted's daughter. It was fashionable in the nineties to use first names only. It was my plan to say his name as often as possible before he arrived the following day. Nothing aggravated me any more than the question, "Does your father know your name?" I always answered, "He doesn't have to; I know my name." I now hoped for compassion and understanding.

My father was assigned to a large, bright and airy room. Along one wall was a large picture window with rose drapery. It pleased me to see that the bathroom area was big enough for patient and nurse to distance themselves from each other and for a nurse to turn her back. Like an overly protective mother I began to fuss up his room. I closed his bedroom door because I knew I was being obsessive when I was lining his bureau drawers. I hung a small black-and-white 1920s photo of my father's dealership on the wall as a conversation piece. I believed the nurses would be looking for something to say to their new arrival and was more than eager to accommodate. It was a topic about which he could still be spontaneous. Later I brought his wingback chair, footstool, and end table and three small labeled family photos. Our daughter Cindy brought a photo album of him with his grandchildren, with a special photo of him and his great-grandson blowing out candles on my father's ninetieth birthday cake. I bought a floor lamp with a very weighted base and hoped for the best, realizing that sometimes Alzheimer patients in their extreme state could pick up and throw an object. I puzzled whether or not to have a full-length mirror in which my father could actually see himself. It was a fascinating question, worth pondering. Would it perk him up, would it help him, or would it shock him and hinder him? He still had a very handsome smile; people still saw him as debonair. He was looked at with the loving eyes of his daughter. But inwardly how was he experiencing himself? *I will bring in my own hand mirror from time to time,* I decided.

I packed his burgeoning wardrobe. I wanted my father to be clean, sweet-smelling. I wanted him to wear modestly the best possible clothes, with plenty of changes. I felt this would help the nurses pay attention to him and, in a special way, love him.

When I returned to the Unit, from out of nowhere appeared a patient with softly padding shoes, looking lost. She wandered in and out of the room opening and closing my father's bureau drawers. Bewildered, I went to the desk to ask if they knew she was missing. I was assured she was just misplaced and that this was normal. I wasn't prepared for this. A few minutes later another woman arrived in his room, completely dressed, with a sweater covering her shoulders, her hair freshly curled, carrying a purse. She approached me and began to pick slowly and meticulously at the fabric on my shoulder. I was scared half to death. For all I knew she might haul off and hurt me badly at any moment. I wondered how to guard myself against someone who was suddenly out of her mind, and why in the blooming world wasn't someone looking after me? After all, they were receiving $200 a day, $6,000 a month, $72,000 a year.

I was reminded of when I went back to college and found myself the only adult in the class. Now once again, like the new kid on the block, I was looking for a helpmate within the system. Her name was Lenna. I watched her changing beds and passing out midmorning juice. I liked her straightforward style. "When you're through with what you're doing, may I help you make up my father's bed?" I asked. I explained to her why we were bringing his own absorbent undergarments. He had been sitting for three years now, and I feared a harsher brand would open up new ulcers. She agreed and suggested we store them in the back of his closet. I had learned earlier that bedsores and ulcers on the buttocks were not to be taken lightly. I asked that someone responsible check his body each week. I had been through a lot already with the

186

nurses and knew that some nurses did a better job than others.

The nursing home had required neurological and psychological testing. I always stayed in the background when we had professional appointments. I didn't want my father's attention to be torn between a well-trained nurse and a well-intentioned daughter. By now Karen had been with us for four years and she and I worked well together. Whatever worked for him was our common goal. She wasn't afraid to tell me why my idea wouldn't work, and I liked that. The goal was to keep his personality on an even keel. He couldn't be rushed, so you wanted to wake him early enough to have his morning coffee and a leisurely breakfast, with enough time left to dress him slowly. This sounds simple, but he was intuitive and could pick up on your plan. Whether it is ethical or not, my father was not the kind of man you lied to. You would never think to tell him he was going out for a ride and end up in the doctor's office; he was worthy of more than that.

Karen got a kick out of being in public with my father. We all did. When you are walking a newborn down the street in a carriage, everyone stops to enjoy this brilliant miracle of life. Being with my well-groomed, well-mannered father was a brilliant miracle of Alzheimer's. Because he was immaculately clean people were comfortable being close to him. You knew by looking at him that he didn't smell. I always made a point of complimenting the nurses when my father looked especially appealing. My father didn't mind waiting rooms because it was his opportunity to "people-watch," but with the anticipation that went along with his being tested, we were glad to be called in right away. Karen and my father sat up front across from the doctor's desk; I sat behind them in the corner. The first question the doctor asked was, "What's your name?"

"Ted Marble," he answered.

Karen seated on the edge of her chair, turned and looked at me with a big grin on her face and with thumb and forefinger pressed together.

Then came the second, more difficult question: "What's your telephone number?"

Karen looked at me and I looked at her. No way would he get this one right. He looked at the doctor straight on and said, "How the hell do I know? I don't call myself." Karen was thrilled! I laughed silently.

The day the psychologist came to the house Karen went through the whole calming process again. Only this time he answered a few questions while seated in his chair and then fell asleep. The lady left. All in all, it was pretty uneventful, and that's the way we liked things.

5

'Twas grace that taught my heart to fear
and grace my fears relieved.
      —"Amazing Grace," Stanzas 1–4,
      John Newton, 1779; alt. stanza 5,
      A Collection of Sacred Ballads, 1790

I hid around the corner in my car when Karen and Gordon drove my father to the Alzheimer's unit. Once I saw them go through the door I left for our rented condominium in Vermont. The two-hour ride up was pleasant and relieving. It felt good to be alone and quiet. I had total trust in both Gordon and Karen. There were too many ambiguities to cry. I was no sooner in the door when Gordon telephoned, "He's there." I could hear his voice crack and a nervous clearing of his throat: "It was the hardest thing I ever had to do in my life." I felt pangs of guilt and quickly justified them away.

The next four days I felt like an exhausted mother. But, after that, there were other feelings. I feared my dear father, even though he was in a unit with forty-two of his peers, was feeling abandoned—his lifelong fear. I telephoned the unit, sensitive about being considered a pest. I always asked to speak to the charge nurse, the most cognizant of the overall picture. I wanted more than just an updated report; I wanted to know how she evaluated my father in the scheme of things. I learned he was friendly and approachable. If a staff member hadn't bought a car at my father's dealership, there was a grandparent, aunt or uncle, or neighbor who had. Whether he recognized them or not, he had a variety of connections with the older visitors through many years of community volunteer work.

On Monday I was back home in Haverhill. My mother had taught me never to visit a hospital before early afternoon, yet my plan was to be at the Alzheimer's unit by 9:00 A.M. sharp. I pulled my car into a parking place close to the building, although usually I park the farthest distance away because walking does me good. Today was different on all levels. My gait was slower than usual.

There came with this situation the fight-or-flight instinct, and I girded my gut and my fiery iron will, and as I pulled myself together the elevator door opened and there he was, seated in a semicircle with mostly women. He looked spit-polished. When I bent down to gently kiss him on the cheek I knew all eyes were on me and that the ladies were being drawn into this loving father-daughter exchange. I realized they loved it! "Hi, Daddy, it's Janet; aren't you glad I'm here? . . . I am."

I could see I was going to be letting go in some ways I hadn't dreamed of before. I was stunned to see Karen walking toward me while assisting another patient. It's one thing to turn my Alzheimer father over to these strangers, but do we need to turn our special duty nurse over, too? Karen immediately pulled me aside. When she arrived at seven o'clock that morning, she had stepped into the bathing room to see my father, hollering and screaming out of fright, hoisted high, in a harness and gradually being lowered into a massive tub. The nurses

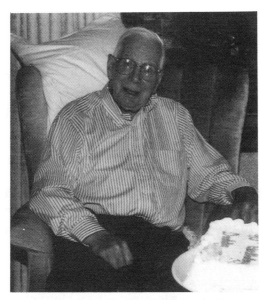

My father on his 90th birthday 1990

meant well, thinking warm water and the jets from the Jacuzzi would relax him after a tumultuous night. What they didn't understand and Karen did, was that my father couldn't swim, nor did he assume strangers to be competent and trustworthy. He was the kind of man who made you earn his respect. Imagine all that commotion when you're already so confused inside? It didn't make sense to me. Karen announced that she's spoken to the nurses at the desk and that she would be giving him his baths on Tuesdays and Thursdays. I smiled in relief.

How can a man be fiery mad in the morning and two hours later be alert and full of finesse? For the next two days Karen and I colluded. With a little wink and a word we understood each other. We learned quickly that there

191

were not only loose cannons on the Alzheimer floor but also lost puzzle pieces. Because not all staff people wore name badges, we had difficulty determining who were patients, staff, volunteers, or visitors. Harriette, for instance, was tall, an erect woman with a pleasant-looking face, and was well groomed. She was one of the regulars who went downstairs every Friday to have their hair washed and styled. Most of her time was spent at the piano, where she played a medley of tunes by ear. She knew most of the words and led the group several times daily in singalongs. I assumed she was a volunteer. It never occurred to me otherwise until Karen came up to me and said, "I think that woman at the piano is a patient." It didn't seem proper at the time to ask the nurses. I didn't want to appear inquisitive. It took another full day of observing to conclude that Karen was right.

I tried to ignore, with little success, the lady sitting with a baby doll in her lap. Without a blanket or a change of clothing, she fussed over it very little. I was relieved to notice how the staff did not encourage regression. When patients went to place their arms around me and I smelled the stench of urine I wanted desperately to pull away, yet I did not want to show my revulsion lest someone be watching. I felt unsanitary and contagious. I wanted to wash my hands all the time, but I couldn't. I waited until I got downstairs and used the ladies' room facilities.

I was shocked the first time I heard the nurse use the word *pee* when asking a patient if she had to urinate. I hoped she wouldn't ask that of my father, especially in front of me. I took baths now even more often, to rinse off the odor of urine from my body and to purify my sense of smell.

Mark Twain tells us, "Wrinkles only say where

smiles have been!" I found it fascinating and wondered all the more at the unwrinkled skin and the childlike eyes. Patients were not holding onto stress in the customary way. Yet Paula hollered all day, every day, continuously. She was filled with intense anger and did not hesitate to strike at anyone in sight. The nurses, alternating in twenty-minute shifts, would walk her back and forth along the corridors, hoping to relieve some of her tension. I was afraid of her but even more of other patients who seemed to be acutely intuitive and might read the fear on my face. I wondered how many potential visitors stayed away due to Paula's behavior. In the old days when I was scared I took a deep breath and tucked in my stomach. I learned now how to simply notice my fear rather than think about it, to focus on my breath and carry a soft belly.

We'd reached the fourth-day mark. Karen dropped in early in the morning and then left the unit to go to her other nursing job. I felt alone and helpless. A man in his midfifties, with a good-citizen-type face, suddenly behaved like a bully looking for trouble. I thought at first it was his way of playing, "Follow the Leader." When I realized that this was no game, I felt I was being hunted to satisfy his violent impulses. Unlike the policeman and the nurse attendant, I had no training. I was terrified. I sensed he felt I was needy and vulnerable. I hesitated to make any sudden moves or to call out to him, "Stop," fearful I would cause other patients to be anxious and they, too, would flare up and suddenly a whole group of Alzheimer patients would be out of control. I knew by then I could fly onto the elevator and out the door, but what kind of impression would I have left? A nurse caught his eye and with great competence sat him right down. I was coming to the realization I would either do something "out of this world" immensely creative, in this environment, or I just could not bear it.

I felt like an outsider in my father's new home, and even though it didn't appear to be true, I feared that he might be feeling the same way, too. When Lauren, the activities director, invited me to join with my father in Group Activities, I thought it best not to refuse. I felt nervous when I learned it was to be held in the room where the less coherent people sat. Intentionally I entered with eyes half-closed. My instincts told me to focus on the environment first and, if I could get through that, then move on to the people present. The room was large and well lit with natural light. The brightly lit aquarium in the corner was sparkling clean. The fish looked healthy and well cared for also. Here and there I saw signs of drool on the floor. I swallowed hard. Off to one side was a craft table. There were as many styles of wheelchairs as there were needs. I was moved to see how well each patient was provided for. Most people were dressed in day clothes. Three women to every man, many women had on brightly colored, washable sweatsuits; others had on dresses and ankle socks. The men wore sweatpants or regular pants and a shirt. Mostly everyone had sneakers on. I felt wretched and ashamed when I paid attention to people's clothes before acknowledging the people themselves. I considered myself a student of Dr. Leo Buscalglia, who for many years taught a popular course at the University of Southern California titled Love, from which originated his successful book of the same name. In this book he encouraged people to think in terms of people before "things."

A strong believer in the power of the subconscious mind, I was glad to see the less aware patients included in the circle of patients. I wanted to understand how my father's condition varied from other patients and what might lie ahead for us. There were those like Harriette who caused me to wonder what she was doing there. Others were unable to hold their heads up straight yet managed somehow to look you in the eye. As repulsive as it was, I tried my hardest to make eye contact. Some looked stiff, as though their bones were at the point of snapping. The more vague they appeared, the more helpless I became. Some spoke with a thick tongue in distorted language that made me feel queasy. Others were simply noncommunicable.

I watched Lauren closely and saw how hard she worked to stimulate and to integrate the patients, through group activity. She recognized my discomfort and tried to help me. I followed her instructions: I walked over to the closet in the corner and took from the carton on the floor an orange ball light as a sponge. She suggested I play catch with my father. The idea was as painful as it was absurd. Although I played catcher in a softball league, I had never played with my father as a youngster. Why in the world would we want to toss a ball back and forth now? Didn't she know it was beyond me to ask him to throw with his deadweight arms? I was his daughter and not his physical therapist. Lauren seemed to take it in stride when I suggested instead to throw the ball to the lady dressed in a jogging suit, wearing a smile.

I abruptly turned and when I did all I could do was stare. There seated in a special kind of chair was a salesman who formerly had worked for my father at the car dealership, he was conscious but not ambulatory and conversant with only a few. I swallowed hard and joined the other guttural sounds in the room. I purposely neglected to tell Lauren, the activity director. I sensed if she knew we shared past history, she'd attempt to drag me over to talk to him, as a stimulant. That's what I'd have done in the same situation. I felt ashamed.

Just as I was about to leave for the day Lauren approached me one more time. "Janet, how would you and your father like to join me and twelve others for a group reminiscence program next Thursday morning at ten." I thought, *Great!* My father and I had been laughing and having good conversation for five years now. We needed new friends and maybe this was just the way to find them. "Thank you," I said. "Karen will be here also."

Especially in my first days at the Unit, I couldn't help but resonate with the dysfunctional around me. A lolling, twisted tongue made my mouth go dry. They took me to their level. I had to find a method to defend myself against my revulsion and terrors in order to shift into creative mode, and I had to do it quickly. Otherwise I might never find a way to climb back out. I realized some people who are not able to eject it out of themselves go home with it and feel ill. It even gives them nightmares.

I found that one of the prime uses of my imagination was pure survival strategy. I had a very ingenious method that included the power of visualization and the feeding of what I liked to call my second mind. Like a warrior I girded myself with a shield. I instructed my second mind to envision a picture of a shield. Through focus and concentration I would live into that image until the protection of the shield felt real. I wasn't just thinking about it; I was doing it. And it worked! I selected the quality of my shield in the morning while getting dressed, the same way I selected the texture of my scarf, on an intuitive level. When I was full of fear and vulnerable I imagined my shield the size of King Arthur's; when I felt strong and confident I needed it only to cover my heart. Like an outfit, I selected my shield for the day. On a good day it was made of thick straw, like an archery target. Another day it might be made of smoky tones or maybe red brick Lucite.

I learned to trust my images and my hunches. There was a time when I believed my strong intuitive flashes were God's whispers and it was my job to be still and listen. Like my father and my mother, I remained fully focused with an iron will on what needed to be done that was positive. This survival strategy allowed me to stay when something was repugnant, to survive the circumstance, and to make a creative contribution all at the same time. Some days when the elevator door opened onto the Alzheimer's floor, I thought I was one footstep away from falling over the edge into a deep, dark hole. If Mae and Harriette were being hot-tempered I feared a fight might break out. Although I'd never seen it happen with my own eyes, I knew it might happen. Paula, full of rage and hollering, was continually pacing the floors. The male wandering minstrel over on the sidelines was looking at me wide-eyed. I reverted to my intuition and imagination, using the analogy of "beyond the rainbow" to picture the dividing line between the Alzheimer world and the outer world. I asked my second mind to help me survive the situation, beyond the fear-and-flight response in the pleasure zone: whimsical and light, the sun is bright, the air smelled clean, and the clouds were a welcoming sight. As I accustomed myself to the Unit, I saw that I wasn't in charge anymore. It both relieved and saddened me. My father would receive extraordinarily good care in an emergency, yet he never again would experience the soothing effect of being in his own home.

My first impulse was to trust all the nurses and to

hold them in very high esteem. It was painful to discover only some were there to serve. I watched the nurses like a hawk. If I saw wobbles in his walk, I made sure he got someone who held him firmly. I was too grateful to be jealous when he had a warm smile for the nurses. At times when they assisted him to his bathroom and he was out of my sight, I sat alone and feared he might never come back or when he did come back he wouldn't be in the here and now.

I began to notice the other family dramas around me. I wondered how I could involve myself with Alzheimer families when in some ways I was neglecting my own. Because of their love for their grandfather, my teenage children were accepting more responsibility. I'd been with them less, and I was not eager to connect to other people who carried the same problem. I connected with the more lucid patients. I discovered my personality seemed to have a good effect on many of the Alzheimer patients.

Every morning when I arrived I would find my father in his semicircle of new friends. Enormously proud of his appearance, I admired his thick white hair perfectly groomed, with nicely pressed shirt and flannel pants. He had finesse and a disciplined demeanor even in the Alzheimer's unit. The way he held his head made him look healthy and cavalier, deceptively in control. He was a work of fine art in the Alzheimer's unit; as if he were a Renoir, people would always stop to look at him. Karen and I sized up all the other men and decided he had no competition. In my view even the dullest person would see that my father was the crème de la crème. With or without his fine attire, his complexion was cared for. His legs were trim, with no bulging veins or ugly sores. He had taken good care of his feet with pedicures once a month and had filed his nails. He was the new male in the neighborhood and up for grabs! I was shocked to see how the female patients, when aroused, competed with one another almost on a barnyard level. Thank goodness he wasn't responding. As his daughter, observing that crude feminine hunger was torture.

One morning I saw a Band-Aid on my father's arm. The nurses told me how the night before he had knocked his arm on the bedrail. I wanted to shriek, "Did you ask him first before raising up the bedrail?" When at home, he refused to have his bed covers tucked in. He was claustrophobic, now they had him caged in. I didn't tell them he was a claustrophic; I assumed I'd be told his safety came first. Reluctantly I learned to recognize the symptoms of his irritable or violent nights. I purposely continued to avoid details. Under the circumstances it was good policy never to ask questions to which I didn't want to hear the answer. The plaid vest restrainer we originally had stored in the bottom drawer of the dining room credenza was now in the bottom drawer of his dresser.

I'd gone nonstop for days on end and was exhausted. I had to secure the house while it remained unoccupied. I was sad when I lost my childhood home to the smell of urine from the bedclothes, but now I was even sadder: my childhood home empty and armored, smelling clean and sweet the way my mother had maintained it. My father's bedding, waste baskets, dish towels, place mats, and napkins were thrown out. I secured a professional cleaning service to come in and wash the downstairs walls, the rugs, even the ceiling light fixtures. They used a special solution to neutralize the scent of urine. I tossed out anything in the bathroom that wasn't nailed down and replaced the toilet seat cover, too. Old lamp shades that smelled stale were replaced. A plumber came to fix two leaky faucets. Gordon had an alarm system installed.

Back in the late 1970s when on my own I had studied the theory of chiropractic I learned how Imhotep, a great physician of ancient Egypt, saw the Nile as a symbol of the "river of life" flowing in the human body. Like life, the real source of the river was a mystery. The Nile, both dependable and unpredictable was like the blood in man, the flow of air in the body of man, the food by which man is sustained. Imhotep pointed out that a stoppage of the Nile's irrigation system brought disaster to the land, thus interference to the channels of the human system worked. I made an agreement with myself to focus my energy toward the healthiest approach. This was my way of demonstrating a positive attitude. My father had lost his mind, his wife, and now his home. I couldn't subject him to losing his daughter, too. Just because my father was in good care now I wouldn't let myself down and get sick. Gordon and the family would have prevailed, but somehow that didn't seem right to me. I was disciplined and willing to do the work. I had already experimented a lot with my headaches. Walking worked, when I did it! An exercise program at the health club aggravated my back, causing me more frequent headaches, even low-impact water aerobics. Meditation helped me get in touch with my soul. Yoga placed added tension on my neck.

I pictured a cup, full of steam, to measure my energy. From this I determined my priorities, using my instincts and intuition as my guide. Two hours of housework, a visit to the grocery store, and a trip to the cleaner's together would equal one quarter-cup. A ninety-minute quality visit at the Alzheimer's unit would deplete the equivalent of nearly a half-cup. On occasion a visit would fill me with such satisfying joy that I was replenished by maybe one-eighth of a cup.

I placed a chair in front of the window and replenished energy from the warmth and the force of the sun. I fed my mind at night by reading from an inspiring book. If I found I was too tired to keep my eyes open or if the emotional stress caused my body to burn and I was unable to concentrate, I'd read chapter titles or thumb through pages for a quote to nourish my soul and to carry me through the next day. Even very close friends could be depleting. I was going to the beach, to the museum, or staying at home to be alone. It was that alone time that replenished my cup. My mode of pure service for so many days, and weeks and months and years was like, in certain ways, that of the religious who give themselves completely to the needs of others. One of the graces of my life is that my creative fire does not go out for long. I thrive on spontaneous, creative activities, and they come relatively easily to me. I found taking care of my parents very different from doing a regular job where I was getting paid.

I wanted my father to sense he was in a family setting and to keep vibrant life happening around him. Each day when the elevator door opened and there he was, seated in the hallway in front of the nurses' station, in a semicircle with four, sometimes five, other patients, I joined them rather than the two of us going off to visit alone. I saw this group as a golden opportunity to unite ourselves with the others; it was a pure creative opportunity.

I elected to sit on the hallway table because of the possibility of urine on the chairs. I thought of my mother, whose feet often didn't quite reach the floor. Swinging my legs back and forth like a child on a picnic bench released my girlish creativity. Yet I didn't know quite what to do. I felt very self-conscious with the nurses seated at the desk behind me. I had set myself the task to continue caring for my father; I sensed the others wanted something to happen for them also. The energy in the group was high; so was my father's mood, I said to myself, *Go for it, Janet. Get some life going for these people, and what better way than to josh around with your father?*

I had developed a perspective on his behavior, and I could tease him about his rigidities when his mind was clear and he could reflect on himself. I began in much the way I had at home. In the old days he was only comfortable with his nose to the grindstone. Nowadays he was an easier sell. In his Alzheimer's the responsible rigidities just melted away, his sense of humor came out of hiding, and he twinkled like a child.

"Daddy, when I was little, you were so ethical, so moral, and had such high standards that you were considered a prude." Where did that come from? I nearly bit my tongue to keep myself from going on.

"Sounds good to me." His boyish smile told me I was on safe ground. The idea was so universal that the people who were sitting around caught the sense of it and howled. This encouraged me more.

"One Saturday afternoon I went to the movies. I know it was Saturday because you didn't allow us to go on Sunday. You said Sunday was family day. Why, you didn't even play golf on that day."

"Is that right?" With the mention of golf I was hoping he was seeing rich green grass.

"Yes, and I got into the theater for underage. I was thirteen and I paid for a twelve-year-old's ticket. My only mistake was in telling you I lied."

"You did that?"

"Yes, I did that. But *you* made me go back and pay the manager the difference."

"Good; I did that right."

He laughed; I laughed; they laughed. It felt good.

Among all the patients, Myrtle held a special place in my heart. She was petite and perky like my mother, depending on what chair she was in, her feet barely reached the floor. One day early on, I heard her chuckle to one of the nurses, "Jesus, Mary, and Joseph, what are you talking about?"

I turned around and laughed out loud, "What, were you and my mother in the same catechism class?"

She shook her head. "Probably."

We bonded from that day on. I followed my intuition. One day when I looked at Myrtle, I saw my mother and I thought, *Garters.* Before I knew it I was off and running.

"Myrtle when you were younger, did you wear garters?"

"Of course I did!" Her sense of timing, her facial expression, made her a stand-up comedian's dream.

"Did you wear the round blue wedding-style garters or those that had hooks?"

"Both." She rolled her eyes as if to say, "Doesn't this girl know anything?"

"So did my mother." But she only wore the round ones on hot and humid summer days. In the winter they were stored in her sewing box.

I looked at Harriette, who had been a physical education teacher and whose father had been a coach at Boston College, of which she was mighty proud.

"Harriette, did you by any chance wear garters to work?"

"Heavens no! You'd never catch me wearing those things. I taught girls' basketball."

203

To me Harriette was the most coherent. Later it was explained by one of the nurses that Harriette was wily, like a fox. She didn't know how to be rational, but she knew how to survive. She spoke in generalities to hide her lack of clarity. She would say, "Isn't that the truth?" or, "You know how it is?" or, "Wouldn't you know?" My father was skilled in that also, as if these phrases soothed people down.

It was pure joy, after years of being a mature and responsible mother to my own family and with my own parents, to now find myself in a childlike role. I was around my father and I sensed that the child part of me would attract them somehow; it certainly had the past five years for him. It also worked for me. If I had been with someone else, the little girl in me who was out to please her father would never have shown up. I would have been far more dignified and introspective. I would have preferred to be quiet and private, share our memories and a few last-minute thoughts, rather than be out gallivanting with others. It would have been just like what my mother said: "Janet, grown-ups don't act that way." I was grateful for the low-key, laid-back people (who weren't getting much done), they balanced out my need for drama. Like a warrior going into battle or a mime performer working the streets, I was able to speak playfully and creatively to the Alzheimer's patients. One early afternoon, after they had just finished their lunch and were feeling lethargic, I took my usual seat at the table. My father had dozed off in the chair next to me. "I want to tell you ladies about the time I went to the health spa and discovered that the grip in my weakest hand recorded stronger than that of the instructor." I gripped my hands and pulled them and they laughed and imitated me and then I knew I was on a good track.

I arrived one day and I had a little waiting time. I noticed a gentleman who had been there every day visiting his wife. It was a melancholy sight to see them holding hands, their heads together whispering. In their sorrow I sensed an aura of dignified peace. I was profoundly envious. Could I create such acceptance for myself? Or would I be too busy fighting by scratching and clawing my way over the rainbow wearing myself down?

I quickly learned not to talk about my children or other family members with the patients because they couldn't follow me. Their loss of the sense of self made it impossible to hear about other selves. I noticed that some visitors were coming into the unit, hopelessly trying to carry on a conversation about individuals to whom the patients had been connected. Because I wanted to get to know these people, I realized gradually that what I needed to do was focus entirely on their sense of enjoyment that was re-creating for them a sense of self and vibrant life. Trained through my relationship with my father, I learned through conversation about the individual's past, and this helped me to elicit more memories. I was trying to gather as much information as possible, so that I could give it back to them at our next visit. I had learned to accept their repetition rather than let myself be unduly irritated by them.

I chose not to dwell in doubts and depression. I viewed the more lucid patients as needy but preferred not to look at them or my father as terminally ill. The well-organized unit with its reliable staff allowed me to maintain my focus and feel safely cared for myself. The patients would drool, mumble, and shuffle. I could safely ignore many of their problems. Sometimes if their behavior began to annoy me I asked, "Do you know how to wink?" They liked this delightful distraction. I could even sometimes be like Mary Poppins, coming in and taking everyone over the rainbow.

In the euphoria of my skillfulness one day I realized some of the nurses were studying me to learn how to have more enjoyment with Alzheimer patients, and I was grateful to be able to share with them. However, I was thinking to myself, *I wonder how long this is going to last. I hope they enjoy it while they have it!*

Some people wear a watch to determine the time. I never did. As the daughter of my father, who was always very precise and regular in his schedules, I had internal clock time at an early age. In those days when I wrote notes to my children, I was in such control that I could even clock my moves to the second. I'd leave notes for my family saying I would be home at 12:22, and that's when I'd be home. So in this way, I was distracting myself from my grief, my loss, and it took me months and months before I could give up my need to control. I was so used to controlling the show, as much as possible, that by the time I reached the Unit I was trying my best not to control. Nevertheless, I wanted all the nurses to take care of my father. Gradually, in my own bizarre way, I thought, *Okay, I'll become extremely competent in taking care of these others so you can take care of this* one. *Because he's the most important to me.*

Elizabeth brought the best out in my father. Unlike the younger nurses, she was able to talk of difficult times such as the depression years. It made him feel comfortable to talk even of the dark old days, she thought. Because his surroundings were new, he liked hearing about familiar things. She worked regularly at a rehabilitation center but was attached to my father and still continued to take afternoon drives to the beach, where they would stop to have dinner. At the entrance door to the restaurant his social habits would turn on and he'd insist she go first, even though she wanted to steady his gait from behind. This gave the impression that he was more in control. He was unable to read the menu but got around that by having Elizabeth order first. Then he'd say to the waitress, "What she just ordered sounds good to me; I'll have the same." Elizabeth told me that years later when she went back they asked for my father and she told them he had died: "They never suspected all the times we went there that he had Alzheimer's. He was a charmer."

Like three jolly elves, on Tuesdays Karen, my father, and I would go out do errands, and one of us would stay in the car with him. A little glance, a little smirk in the rearview mirror, and Karen and I understood each other. Determined to have as much fun as we could, we'd go for fast food to make his nose wriggle until we opened the bags back at the Alzheimer's unit.

My father had been a man conscious of his shoes, choosing them with great fanfare. He changed them in the middle of the day in order to refresh his feet. When the staff suggested sneakers my heart sank, because he had never worn them. Worriedly I let the nurses in on my feelings. I saw there was little room for compromise and their reasoning was valid. The sole of the sneaker grips the floor, making it less likely for him to fall and easier for him to move from a seated to a standing position. He pleasantly surprised me by taking to sneakers like a duck to water. "Best shoes I've ever owned," he said with a twinkle. I had been warned earlier that other patients treated others' clothes as if they were their own. I was finding other people's things in his closet, yet his were never missing. I wondered why no one showed any interest in wearing his wardrobe.

A woman in the unit always wore dresses with white nylon knee-high stockings. One day I found myself curious whether she was wearing her underwear, the same way a child is who picks up a doll to see if she clothed underneath. Then I thought, *Wait a minute; would you please put your legs together?*, but she didn't. My next thought was, *If she doesn't have her underpants on, should I call a nurse?* I realized then how vigilant the nurses had to be to keep everyone appropriately clean and clothed.

When sad emotions clouded my thoughts, rather than respond to them I simply let them go. One day I was told that because of my father's repetitive late-night mumblings the nurses had transferred him to another room, as he was too disruptive to his roommate. His new roommate, Fred, was stone deaf. It pained me deeply to find my father had become a sociable, well-intentioned listener during the day, a silent outcast at night.

It was Thursday, Karen's day to be with my father and the day we were to observe Lauren. The three of us followed the whole group into the sun parlor for her weekly reminiscence program. In the past I had studied the flocking patterns; now I was learning the flocking patterns of patients and how they followed the leader like a flock of lost sheep. Karen sat next to my father, but I sat across to help center him. The warm exchange between Lauren and her patients pleased me. It was clear to see she cared about these people and genuinely liked them. She began her program by talking about the neighborhood iceman who once hauled blocks of ice into everyone's kitchen. This brought back vivid memories for me, and I eagerly joined in on the conversation. We talked in descriptive terms first: On my street the iceman's truck was green; on others it was blue. Most of the activity went on in the back of the truck, where the iceman lifted a brown rubber bib that covered his shoulders, then grabbed his giant tongs. He never left the curb without chipping away at an ice block until a chunk broke away, then handing us ice chips that felt cold and wet in the hand and freezing cold to the lips. Although my memory of the iceman was clear, I had no recollection of the icebox. I was amazed that some of the Alzheimer's people had more vivid and precise memories than I did.

It was not my style to hold back but instead to lead people on. So, when quiet, expressionless Eleanor said to me, "Do you know my Uncle Fred?" I said, "I'm not sure, maybe! Tell me more about him."

"He has a driveway like this." She made a semicircle motion with her hand.

"Oh! A wraparound driveway. Is his house that big one with all the green lawn?" I hoped they'd forgive an innocent lie. It didn't matter, because what was important was the sharing.

"Very big," she answered.

My intuition tapped in, again, in grand style. "Does he have a big belly, too?" She hesitated; I hopped to it. Otherwise I would have lost my audience. "Yes, I do know Uncle Fred. As a matter of fact, I saw him last week, downtown. He had his nose pressed up against the bakery window, staring at the Bismarcks."

"He always ate too many of those."

I had them laughing as a group.

After observing Lauren's session with great admiration, I walked out of the room thinking, *I can do that, too!*

I began to sense that I needed to go on sharing all that had come to me in my love and care of my father. I, too, knew how to be with Alzheimer patients! It was unthinkable not to share it. I had discovered a very constructive way for me to distract myself from my distress. I'd grown accustomed to some of the patients while visiting with my father in the foyer, but I was looking to stretch myself to come even more alive.

After a week of swinging my legs and attending Lauren's group, I felt moved enough and confident to ask if I could run a weekly session during the week. I had learned to trust Lauren the most when I was confused or dismayed or frightened by the behavior of the patients. She seemed to have an intuitive understanding of my passionate need to serve my father and was willing to get out of the way. She also compassionately understood my need to be active and what a suffering it was for me to have to be an observer. I had noticed early on that she was deeply interested and respectful of the entire extended family. I was moved that she sacrificed her role as group leader. With her sense of clinical responsibility she agreed to let me run the group, but she would observe and be sure that everything went right. She always stayed with me in the room.

As an activities director Lauren was never given the esteem that nurses and doctors received, although she did deserve it. I didn't know Lauren's story, but by intuition I knew we had a deep understanding and an appreciation of each other with few words said. We knew right away that our understanding of how to work with Alzheimer patients was similar. We both realized it was essential that they were up and dressed in the morning on schedule, that they have physical movement, and that they have regular periods of active stimulation for their memories as well and to go with them wherever they went with a sense of fun and respect. It takes a lot of faith in them that they deserve respect for what capacities are left in them and that they should be able to function as well as possible. We shared a willingness to be surprised by sudden functionings that were unexpected and were willing to watch for those moments. We were both tolerant of individual differences, and we even enjoyed that they were at different levels of functioning.

It was difficult entertaining my father, but it was twelve times more difficult with a group, and certainly in the beginning. I knew as a volunteer working for the Unit I was covered by insurance, but Lauren's presence helped to ease any other impending fears. Karen's presence helped to ease my fears, too, should my father show signs of jealousy and begin to act out. At home he had showed jealousy towards my mother with the nurses; he never expressed that emotion with me here.

I had developed a lot of clinical clarity. I was inspired and I was self-taught. I also had taken credited therapy courses in Boston and attended conferences that taught me the performance side of storytelling.

I always dressed to look my best when going to visit my parents. But now my drive to make myself look, "just right" was growing even stronger. By tending my appearance, I could better handle all the chaos in the Unit. I felt more in control. I have since learned that this is not unusual with anyone who is going into difficult situations. While I was selecting my clothes I was also tuning up my integrity. I selected my clothes on an intuitive level and not by the temperature outside. It became extremely important to me not to feel disjointed but rather to feel whole when entering the Alzheimer unit. Anything lively, colorful, and exaggerated tended to hold their attention and to gear me up. I wore creative outfits, storyteller's clothes, long dresses and long light, colorful scarves for drama. The scarves symbolized for me the way Alzheimer disease caused the patients to float in and out themselves. I never wore bracelets or perfume. Little things distracted me and them. I did wear dangling earrings, thinking they framed my face and enhanced my expression. Some days I added extra color to my cheeks to have them appear more childlike. I paid particular attention choosing my shoes, knowing some of the women had worked in local shoe factories. In the winter I wore low-calf laced button boots, a style that had come around again. Myrtle, the one who reminded me of my mother, called them Mary Poppins shoes. Most of the time I wore penny loafers, and they got a kick out of those, particularly when I put shiny new dimes in the openings.

With each visit as I stepped off the elevator I made certain I had removed my sunglasses and replaced them with my bifocals. I had developed the habit of checking my glasses while visiting my parents at their home for the past six years. There was no use in my looking into their eyes to keep them centered if they were unable to see mine. I always chose a wooden chair rather than an upholstered leather one, as it had less stench and allowed me to move more easily. I was orderly in my conversation. As I had trained for so long, with my father, I knew what to do. I sat very erect and totally focused myself. To keep their attention and my concentration my eyes could not divert; my feet could not fidget. I enunciated clearly, I exaggerated my entire being. My whole self was in the service of that little spark of healthy life that I could find and generate. If I had lost the focus that they needed, I said their names to keep them grounded. The more tension I pressed on them the more they were able, it seemed to me, to press back. I think of this now when I hold my two-month-old grandson's bare feet in the palm of my hand. I apply a little pressure, and he bends his knees and pushes back. The more I pressed, gently but firmly, the more the Alzheimer patients released their memories. I was fascinated and delighted again and again.

I learned not to expect more than a three-sentence response from them to a question I had plucked out of my intuition. Lower-functioning people would say three or four words and I'd fill out their sentence. Once in touch with something very meaningful to them, sometimes they were able talk quite normally for a little while.

I would expect the best and I'd get it, the same way other people who expected the worst got that, too. Classic studies in the classroom have shown that children who are expected to become brilliant and the children who are looked at as being incapable and stupid tend to become that. I wonder if anyone has made that kind of study in an Alzheimer's unit. Now, in retrospect, I see what a wonderful field of research this could be. Their intuition was strong, and it got stronger.

When I was a child my father told me, "If you pay attention to the small things, the big things will take care of themselves." Now at the Alzheimer's unit I had a knack for making the biggest thing out of something small. I'd bring in props from my mother's attic to use as stimuli. I carried the objects in a burlap satchel that had a jolly bag-lady image imprint on both sides of it. Years back, one Christmas, my son, Jeffrey, had given it to me as a joke. Laundry and housekeeping held a position of respectability within the neighborhood in the old days. Airing of blankets, various-styled clotheslines, even clothespins and clothespin bags made for busy conversation. One day I brought in my Mother's homemade root beer paraphernalia and spoke about the cool, dark area underneath our cellar stairs where she stored the quart bottles during the hot summer months. This brought great response! Cellar memories for many of the patients also were poignant—the delicious damp smell of the basement, the earthy colors of the vegetables. When they spoke of wooden barrels stored in the basement, filled with potatoes, winter and acorn squash, and onions, I added, "I thought wooden barrels were meant only to store pickles." I enjoyed learning from them. "Ladies, that cobalt blue bottle my mother had sitting on top of the shelf over her washtubs, was that for the laundry or was that the blue rinse she used for her hair?"

The more adapted I became at the Unit, the more accustomed I became to the wanderers. Their weaving in and out was not an issue when we were seated in the lobby; other patients paid little attention, particularly when there was little else going on in their lives. But now in these sessions they were opposed to any dark clouds moving in on their parade. When one of the wanderers began to walk in on us it was like sitting in the grandstands at Fenway Park in Boston: "Sit down. Hey, you there, sit down. Can't you see she's talking?" Then someone else would get annoyed at the person hollering and start shadow-punching her in the ribs.

I had been observing various kinds of humor for many years. I didn't like slapstick. I loved hilarity, a special brand of humor that does not harm and lifts one up. I knew I could achieve it, if I just paid attention. In Isaac Asimov's book *Treasury of Humor* he points out what makes something funny. One of the qualities is that you have an expectation of one thing and then you go the other way. The difference is so extraordinary that you fill that space with laughter. I always assumed taking hilarity in the midst of this very sad situation. We often were surprised by laughter and the vitality and pleasure it released.

One of the reasons I was so successful was because I went right to nitty-gritty, funny pockets of experience. With some of the patients a naughty reminiscence was what gave them the greatest delight: "Now, Myrtle, we all know you liked men! Trust me; that's fine." First she blushed, then fanned her face with her hand.

"You can't fool us, Myrtle. Any lady who put her heart and her soul into organizing USO dances had to like men. Why, you must have been the talk of the town." Those who were alert roared, and the others, I liked to think, were inwardly smiling. Myrtle, still blushing, smiled shyly.

"Myrtle, did you own a red taffeta dress?"

"Yes. How did you know?"

"Because all of us either did or wished we did." I forged on. "Remember the swish-sounding noise the taffeta made when you walked? It made me feel so grown-up and ladylike, the same way stepping into high heels for the very first time did.

"Myrtle, did you wear one of those itchy crinolines underneath your dress, to make it stick out far?"

"We all did." I wanted to think, by the twinkle I saw in her eye, she was seeing and feeling the dress in her mind. I know I was. My intuition was working overtime today.

"I have a question for you, Myrtle, and we're looking for the truth. Were you one of those girls, like Hollywood's Mitzi Gaynor, who danced on top of the tables?"

"Good grief, no!" she said with a zing in her voice. "Well, maybe only once or twice."

The Thursday following her wedding, I brought in our daughter Valerie's gown, the same gown I had worn at my wedding. The full-length taffeta gown had a cathedral train with a fitted bodice outlined with Alencon lace. Bands of embroidered lace extended down the front of the skirt and the entire length of the skirt and train in the back. I decided to put the veil on my head, which was delightful for me and astonishing for the patients. I demonstrated for them the lifting of the veil, all the time trying to put into words the experiences of being a bride and being at a wedding. I overcame my embarrassment at the nurses looking in because I hoped that this would be a luxuriant moment for the patients. It was. All my movements were intentionally quiet and slow. I wanted them to have a moment to raise up their memories in their own time. We gathered in a circle, spreading the lace train in a large semicircle until it covered all our laps. I felt some marriage memories might be difficult, so I chose to focus on the skill of making the dress and having it in the family. I drew their attention reverently to the feel of each detail as we gently ran our fingers across the pearls and softly traced the patterns of lace. I wanted to evoke not only sense memories but also the feeling memories. I spoke now and then. I was glad that they could truly be in touch with beauty and skill and celebration of love and joy.

Tom, a former navy man, liked being made accountable for the times he was caught with his hand in the cookie jar. He seemed lost in thought, and the next I knew, we were talking about cigarettes and beer. I got a lot of my clues from my memory of movies or, in Tom's case, from old newsreels at the theater, back in the days when they had double features.

"Tom, when you were stationed in the service, didn't you serve on a boat?"

"It wasn't a boat; it was a ship! The *U.S.S. Constitution.*" So be it.

"But didn't you also like to smoke?"

"All the time I smoked." The confidence in his voice touched me.

"Tom, I've never been in the service and I certainly was never stationed on a ship, but I know darn well it was against the rules to smoke. Let us in on it, Tom; where did you light up?"

"Downstairs, next to the boiler room."

"What brand did you smoke, Tom?" By now he's laughing hard and the rest of us are enjoying this raw male motif.

"Camels, of course," he replied with a big grin on his face.

"Is that where you had your beer, too?"

"You've got it!" He guffawed, slapping his leg.

I looked at Ruth and saw a young society girl. I found myself thinking of the classic *The Great Gatsby.* I turned to her and said, "When you were young and sat in the back, in the rumble seat of a car, did you hold hands with your beau?" Myrtle roared. The rest of us sat silent waiting for the answer. "Come on, Ruth," I said. "You can tell us. We're all too old for it to matter." She smiled bashfully but was too overwhelmed to reply. "That's OK, Ruth; your silence is golden with us."

I didn't have a card and my role wasn't formalized in any way. So unless people were good and sensitive observers, they didn't have a lot of clues as to who I was and what I was doing. Sometimes, to my bewilderment, visitors came in when I was doing a program and tried to understand what was going on. At first I felt ashamed, that I

217

wanted total control and because of that I was being pos-
sessive and selfish. When I relaxed and eased up on myself I remembered how important it was for the patients
to have limited stimuli in order not to shut down. Every
now and then the nurses and aides dropped in just to sit
down to get a load off their feet. I thought they were in-
truding on our play time. This often had an inhibiting effect. I lost energy. When they started to chat, the fire
coming out of my nostrils got horns and a tail. I felt in-
sulted. They treated my program as casual entertainment for themselves.

Helen didn't like being drawn into the reminiscence
program, even though she liked it once she was there. The
staff encouraged her to attend. Helen had worked in Boston and had spent her lunch hours shopping the business
districts. No stranger to that area, as early as grade
school I would take the train into the city with my mother
and shop for my new fall coats. I expanded on those
memories. One day I spoke about the grand production of
purchasing leather gloves. I vividly mimed trying on
gloves at R. H. Stearns on Tremont Street, pushing the
imaginary leather down over my fingers. They imitated
my tactile gestures, stimulating their own memories,
whether they could articulate them or not.

All the time my father was alive I went to the Unit
five days a week, and when I wasn't doing a formal group
I was swinging my legs on the table in the hallway, working informally to the best of my ability. The truth is I was
struggling to find my role and at the same time I was creating my role. Sometimes I was the vulnerable daughter;
sometimes I was the dynamic entertainer; sometimes I
thought I was housemother going into the college dormi-
tory and looking after the students. Harriette, the piano
player, liked to shake hands with people, and when she

had a hangnail it troubled her. I'd go to the desk and ask if someone could please manicure her nails. Then I'd check back later on in the day. Lauren mentioned one day that Myrtle was finding it uncomfortable to wear earrings; apparently the clips were too tight. I hustled back the next day with two pair of my mother's foam rubber backs. When I had a concern about one of the patients, I'd ask Lauren if we could speak about it in her downstairs office. She was always grateful for my perception.

I was very sad when Lauren called me down to her office to tell me that due to cutbacks, she was going to have to leave. I was astonished that they let such a well-qualified activities director go. With all the more determination I decided to continue the group. As long as I was doing my job, they weren't going to cut me back, because they didn't pay me anything. Now that I was alone the nurses checked upon me many times and saw what I was doing. The sun parlor doors still remained closed, but I sat in view of the nurses' station. I felt disrespected when the nurses let a wanderer walk in on a group, because it took all of my power to maintain the focus for the group participants. I regret that I did not know how to express my anger and frustration to the nurses. Gradually I learned to let my anger go when I was forced to deal with wanderers.

My prayer life was strong. Although I wasn't going to the minister or to confessional, I oftentimes drove to St. John's Church, one quarter-mile down the street. It was there I did my crying and asked God for strength. I prayed also to be understood. Outwardly I had it together; inwardly I was crumbling in despair. At the Girls Club I was altruistic. Now my altruism was all focused on one person. There were benefits in it for me: I loved being onstage, I had control of the audience, and I wasn't going to be judged, nor was I going to judge myself. It was an ironic pleasure for me to find an environment where I could feel safe, liked, and respected at the same time, after all the stress of feeling like a caretaking outsider at home. Gradually the patients became a kind of adjunct family for me, and I adopted them, and to the best of their ability they adopted me. They forgot who I was, yet we felt connected, through my father.

Mae had a special fondness for men, something that I could relate to. She was less animated than the rest but seemed to be more in touch with her heart. She had grown up just outside of Boston and in Vermont, where she spent wonderful summer hours fishing with her elders. She had married a man who played in a band and followed him on his weekend gigs. I was touched when she said, "They were all very good to me." The day I did a program on the big band sounds, she became the leader and the orchestra, all wrapped up in one. Tommy Dorsey was her favorite. We relied on her to fill in the words when we were at a loss. I learned the day I brought in a collector's book on nursery rhymes that she was skilled at remembering them, too.

I discovered that music seemed to be mysteriously untouched by the devastation of Alzheimer's. Each week I brought in four or five pieces of sheet music from my mother's piano seat, which we had moved to the front hall of our house. Seeing her handwritten name in each corner made me feel closer to her. We began and ended each session with a verse of "Oh! What a Beautiful Morning." They loved to emphasize the, "Oh-h-h-h-h-h," as if we were at summer camp. We sang other songs, like "For He's a Jolly Good Fellow" and "Just Another Polka." I chose songs with playful words, "Lavender Blue Dilly

Dilly" and "Bell Bottom Trousers." We sang holiday songs, too: "Easter Parade" and "Yankee Doodle Dandy." I didn't know all the words, so they'd lead me. It gave me joy to give them back some control. When Mae and Harriette would like four-and five-year-old girls say, "Shut up," to each other, I ignored it! Most of the others did, too. Some had lost everything, even the ability to hang onto their own urine. Sitting there surrounded with twelve Alzheimer people, who by now were not patients but instead my friends, was painful and sad.

After meditating on it for a week, I decided to sing "Now is the hour, that we must say good-bye, soon we'll be sailing far across the sea, while you're away oh, please remember me." It was another way for me to validate their feelings. It turned out to be a good choice on my part. After that, now and again, I would bring in a melancholy tune and trust it.

As I continued to tune into their memories and help them to resurface in an enjoyable way, one sunny day we got to talking about their trips to the beach. In a burst of enthusiastic imagination I couldn't resist asking, "Were all your bathing suits black and did they all come down to the knees?" I was genuinely curious. Some stared at the wall; I think I heard someone gulp. At any rate, I didn't get much of an answer. I forged ahead. I wanted them to smell the sea air again, to feel the sand on their feet, and to watch the gulls fly overhead. As ever, I tried to bring about as much delight and laughter and enjoyment as I could. I turned to Jane and noticed her white hair had been freshly done and her skin was smooth, her expression serene. Like my mother often did in her dozing years, Jane sat upright in her chair with her eyes closed. I felt it was her way of keeping her thoughts to herself, her life private, and the nurses at a distance. Just in case Jane

221

was not trying to avoid the world but rather waiting for something to happen that she could relate to, I asked, "Were there large beach areas in Canada?"

Her answer was matter-of-fact: "I never went to the beach; I just worked."

I'd heard answers like that before, from my father. Rather than be uncomfortable with it, I probed further, "What was it like back then to be poor?"

I sensed her relief when she answered, "We had three pairs of shoes for five children and took turns staying home from school. Winter or summer we wore the same clothes. My mother canned a lot, so we always had plenty of food." The more I learned how hard Jane had worked, the more I admired her beautiful robust hands. I prayed over her hands the day I heard she was dying.

I was raised in a house where hands were appreciated. There was always a dispenser of lotion on the counter by the sink, and both my parents used it. My father was one to manicure his own hands. My mother's nails were professionally polished. As she became older and her fingers were disjointed I marveled that she was able to maintain exquisite penmanship. Now I watched my own hands at work with the same intensity and joy that children watch puppets with. When they hurt I believed it was because they were tired of giving. I began to carry hand cream around in my car. Before entering and after leaving the Unit I would massage, individually, each finger. As I woke up to my hands, I began to have manicures. I found it soothing to have them soak in warm water. I didn't like it when a professional massaged them. Revved up and uneasy, I feared the soothing strokes might slow me down. My hands were like precious jewels to me, and I didn't want them covered with extra fingerprints. I was very hesitant about touching patients, yet one day I was moved to feel the coolness of the silk blouse Jane was wearing. I felt impelled to say, "Jane, did you ever think the day would come when you'd be dressed in silk?" She opened her eyes and looked at me—they were as clear as a bell: "No, I never thought I would."

Jim Bradley, a member of our church, liked to tell me of the old days when he lived in the square next to my father's garage. Jim and his pals took old oil cans my father left by the side of his building in the alley, waiting to be picked up. They rested them on two wooden horses with one can dripping into another: "That's how we got oil for the chains on our bikes." Every person there had lived through the days of the depression, and I new on some level that they could relate. My father liked the story and listened like an alley cat with a grin on his face. Struggles come with a sense of accomplishment. It was healthy, I thought, to bring to them a sense of positive resolutions. Mae, the woman who had a warm heart toward men, had been a hardworking waitress at the Sheraton Hotel in Boston. She took childlike pride in telling us how Speaker of the House Tip O'Neil would always ask for her: "He was a good tipper too."

One spring day I thought how invigorating it would be to share old-fashioned games with the group. That Tuesday I stepped off the elevator, full to the brim with glee, like Kate Smith coming out from behind the gold curtain. Lights, action, and urine. . . . "When the moon comes over the mountain. . . ." I pulled first from my pillowcase a black-and-red scatter rug designed to look like a checkerboard, with jumbo-sized checkers to match, and placed it on the floor. Their response was greater than what I had imagined. I don't know if it was the size of the rug, the contrast in colors, or the warm memory of playing the game, but they were smiling and eager to respond when I asked, "What move shall I make next?" After scaring them half to death by plucking bubbles out of the air, I decided on a Chinese-style jumprope, one that rests on the floor, rather than the traditional-style one that swings in midair. I began to recite jingles like, "A my name is Alice, my husband's name is Albert, we come from Alabama, and we sell apples. B my name is Barbara . . ." To my surprise, Mae began to pick up where I left off. It was fun going back to a time when child's play was still kid stuff, playing hopscotch with chalk and making nice big jumps and turnabouts. As I sat on the floor with my skirt tucked in between my legs playing jacks, pickup sticks, and marbles, I could see my mother looking down and hear her saying, "Jesus, Mary, and Joseph, she's still at it."

One day I brought in the contents of my mother's sewing basket. I thought they could enlighten me on a few articles, such as her darning ball and another small, flat, tinny mystery item. They told me it was used to thread needles. I asked them to show me how. I handed it to Margaret; she was the real seamstress. When the nurse came through the door and saw her Alzheimer patient with needle and thread in her hand, I feared I might be fired from my nonpaying job. Nevertheless, all went well.

One day I had seen on Lauren's desk, *Reminisce, the Magazine That Brings Back the Good Days,* for a resource list. I went to the library and pulled forth from it other program ideas. The warm personal memories were so rich and entertaining that eventually I took out a subscription for myself and gave others as gifts. It helped me evoke seasonal events: picnics, watermelon feasts, celebrations and fireworks in July and in the fall apple picking, raking leaves, and going back to school. On days when, as a group, the energy was down, I'd draw on more general topics—the old-time phone company and its hometown operator. I'll never forget the look of surprise on my father's face when I recited for him his old four-digit home and business phone numbers. Old radio programs were another popular topic. My memory of those was foggy, but Gordon's was clear. We also talked about washing machines and midget racers.

One day I unwittingly blew multitudes of soap bubbles and remembered, too late, how just one balloon had made my father frantic. I had no sooner put the child-size wand to my lips when I realized I'd made a big mistake. I jumped up from my chair and began to pluck the bubbles one by one, out of the air. No sooner did they see it when it was gone. This confused them even more. I discovered how quickly fear could be stirred though the senses as well as the pleasures.

I knew that women of my parents' generation had used cold cream and thought how nice it would be for them to experience that familiar smell once again. If their sense of smell had deteriorated, perhaps the memory of the scent could be keen. I remembered how Gordon's grandmother raved when I brought some for her. I was hoping here it might be the same. There were twelve people lined up along the walls. I asked them first to cup their hands. Those who could did. I started with Harriette because she was more alive in her fingertips, though skittish. The amount of cream I used was less than a dime. It had barely reached her hand when she snatched it away. I'm still not certain what caused her fright, the cold, wet sensation of the cream or seeing a foreign substance in her hand. Either way, I was surprised to see how strong her sense response was. I changed my tactic and rubbed it on the backs of the other people's hands, and for those who didn't want any, I placed my hand under their nose and satisfied their sense of memory that way. So when I saw Harriette with fear in her eyes, my first thought was, *How do I regain her trust and that of others who might well have been experiencing the same fear?*

I had learned from my father how easily an Alzheimer patient can be overstimulated. I knew that the distraction of television and radio altered the energy in the room while he was already deeply engaged in confusion. He couldn't tolerate it unless it was for a brief period of time and something concrete, like the six o'clock news, which provided topics of conversation. One day a nurse suggested we buy a VCR for my father's entertainment; needless to say, I discouraged the idea. I wanted him to be connected to a candid, compelling moment that was happening and not a canned moment that was taking place over there in that box or in that radio. Later when my father was at the Unit and I would arrive to find him and other patients on the porch dozing with the television on, I asked to have it turned off. They awoke and something else began to happen because I was really there interacting with them.

Every now and then I'd come down the elevator and look in the dining room. All twelve of the high-functioning patients in my group would be seated around tables. I knew the time we had spent upstairs was lost. I had no illusions about that. Yet because they were used to enjoyment and laughter when I was there, now when they saw me some of them were like pups wagging their tails in delight, which showed me I had really reached them and gave me a surprising sense of satisfaction.

My role at the Alzheimer's unit was very complex. I was calling people my friends who were out of their minds. I sensed that the dying process with this disease

226

had a purpose that I did not yet understand. Something was lifting me onto a spiritual plane, raw and contradictory as it was. I kept Rumi on the bedstand and Kabir in the kitchen but could not find time to read either poet. It was as though the rainbow had come down to meet me rather than my climbing up to reach it one Thursday at my regular program time. There were only women present. Later I saw it as a blessing. For days I'd been mulling over the women of their era. Like a sudden burst of fireworks lit up, I placed my lap harp on the floor and put the pick in my blazer pocket. I spoke in earnest, the same way I'd speak to members of the United Nations: "Ladies, you know how ordinarily we speak of old memories and fun times?" Some nodded yes; others just stared! "I want to talk today on a more serious nature. There is something very important I think you should know about." By the look in their eyes and their degree of concentration I knew I was getting through to them. "There is a rumor going around all across the world. People are saying that someday soon, maybe within ten years, the United States of America is going to have a woman president." I couldn't believe what came next! They actually began to clap and cheer, "Yeah!", first one and then another. I got goose bumps! I'd seen them on numerous occasions act out in a group response, but never with this intensity. "Wait; I haven't told you yet the most important part of all." The room became unusually quiet; even those who ordinarily were in a minitrance were now wide-eyed and looking in my direction. "The reason why we'll someday have a woman president is because of women like you. How did you do it? How did you wait on your men hand and foot and manage to raise strong daughters, all at the same time? Remember how you would place your husband's slippers next to his chair at night before he arrived home from work, and how you would never dream of serving him anything other than a hot meal for dinner, even in the summer when it was ninety-nine degrees in your kitchen?" Their heads were bobbing "yes." I knew I'd reached them on an emotional level, but somehow I wanted more, if only for myself. "Let's hear it, ladies! Three cheers for women! Hip, hip, hooray!" I threw my right arm high in the air with an outstretched hand; they followed it with their eyes. The second time I threw my arm up first, they joined in with bravado. With the third "Hip hip hooray!" those who could were lifting their arms in the air.

Suddenly I felt a tug on the sleeve of my left arm. I looked down to see a small, quiet woman looking up at me with a big grin on her face, "I wish I could get my arm as high as yours," she whispered.

With a grin as big as hers, I answered, "Your arm is already as high as the sky!"

It was essential I find a way to put myself back together again after an encounter with a whole group of dysfunctional people I was trying to "fix" when they couldn't be fixed. I had enough fire and determination to be able to keep that up quite a long time, but by the end of the hour I was exhausted. I always rode the elevator down alone, even if it meant having to wait. I changed back into my sunglasses before the door opened and I stepped into the lobby. I went to wash my hands. Once in the car I'd sit quietly with my hands in repose and let all the pent-up energy pour out of my body. Then I'd either go to the church, or drive to the car wash to cool down, or pick up lunch at a nearby variety store, tempted to buy a bag of soft candy and scoff them down, but instead I settled for feta cheese on my salad. Then I would go home a

228

basket case until, once again, the fire reignited in my belly.

I had been training myself to live in the moment. Every moment has a beginning, middle, and end. It had its own innate value. I was glad that I could create laughter and twinkles. In addition to that, it was distracting me from my sadness and helplessness. I was totally in the service of my father as part of my devotion to him. It was my filial deep love and responsibility to give him the best possible life that he could have, on principal, to create as good an environment as I could possibly make it, in every possible way. That had been my dedication all along, and I just kept it up. I found great purpose in doing this work for others. There was a real soul-satisfying sense of making a contribution, of spiritual merit, of shifting the whole world a little bit by attending to something that needed to be attended to.

It was Tuesday, May 19, 1992, in the early afternoon. I was at the Unit for the second time that day, swinging my legs on the table in the foyer in the midst of our mock-family circle. I noticed many changes from my first visit over a year and a half ago. Myrtle had grown more petite and less feisty yet still wore her earrings and reminded me of my mother. In contrast Harriette didn't look a day different, although she was playing the piano less frequently. Helen was now vague and one of the wanderers. Tom was incoherent and sat in the room on the left. Sitting next to me, in good humor, was still the *crème de la crème,* my father. The Unit was relatively quiet, which was customary, that hour of the day. Shirley, the nurse, was busy with paperwork at the nurses' station. I'd grown much less self-conscious with the nurses.

"Daddy, let me tell you what a wonderful job I felt you did in raising me."

He turned and grinned. "Sounds good to me."

I began slowly, then gained momentum. As usual, I felt embarrassed, yet filled with total determination to let him know his accomplishments. "Daddy, when I was young, in my teens, and you spotted me slumped in a chair, in your special authoritative kind of voice you'd say, 'Sit up straight; look alert.' Now here I am in my fifties, sitting up straight, on time, and no slouch."

Harriette echoed before he had a chance to reply, "Looks good to me."

At a time in his life when his daily routine had little substance, it seemed appropriate to quote back to him some of his words of wisdom. "Daddy, someone asked you once, if you had your life to live over, what would you do different? You answered, 'Instead of always being twenty minutes early I'd plan instead to be right on time. I wasted too much time waiting for others.' I learned a great lesson in that from you, Daddy."

His broad grin made him look healthy and proud, momentarily satisfied. "I did do good work, didn't I," he said.

That evening Gordon was at a baseball game and I was at home. My father died at age ninety-two of a massive heart attack on his way to have a little cut mended at the hospital. I made sure that Gordon had taken off his coat when he got home before I told him. Despite everything, my father's death was unexpected. The following day when I went back to distribute some of his belongings there was no question but that many of the patients also were grieving and that we were all experiencing the loss together. When I gave the nurses my gratitude, Shirley, in her soft-spoken voice, told me when she heard of my father's death what first came to her mind was the conversation he and I had had that final afternoon: "How many of us wish, too late, to let someone know how wonderful we are because of them." To this day I continue to refer to them as my Alzheimer friends, who helped me in my grief and in my sorrow those last days, those last months, and the last year of my father's life.

For the past six years my father had led a quiet life. We held a quiet private funeral. His blind friend, Charlie Hurwitz, gave the eulogy.

Epilogue

When I think back I am fascinated by the way my relationship with my parents opened up and changed during their dying years. Since my parents' death I have continued to grow. Seven years have passed since my father's death. Although I have not fully recovered from the continual unpredictability of my father's disease, during this time I have been able to develop broader vision and to grow spiritually and emotionally.

I continued in the Alzheimer's unit for a year and a half. After my grieving eased, there was a hiatus, and then again I felt the need to do something extraordinary. I decided one day the choicest way to put myself and my experience to the best possible use was to write. Through friendship and professional consultation I have gained much new perspective and well-won freedom from the patterns that were driving me at that time. People sometimes say to me, "Has it been cathartic to be doing this writing?" and I say to them, "I have discovered some of the feelings that were driving me at that time. I needed to grieve for myself and develop a perspective on how obsessive I was. In that sense it has been cathartic. Yet not because I had to grieve for my parents more; I was doing that all along and very deeply."

There was a time I struggled with the thought, *Do I have Alzheimer's?* I journaled because I needed to take hold of my growing insecurity. Finally I got rid of this fear and I said, "I don't know if Alzheimer's is or isn't hereditary; I'm not an expert. I only know I didn't get my father's penis, so why should I assume I'll inherit his disease?"

I now fish with my husband and my grandchildren, and perhaps someday when this book is published I will create a rock garden. I still resist reading articles on Alzheimer's disease. Yet I look forward to sharing my experience with others who are experiencing this devastation. The writing has been good for me.

Bibliography

Books I kept by my bedside back in 1986:

Maltz, Maxwell. *Psycho Cybernetics*. New York. Simon & Schuster, 1960.

Murphy, Joseph. *The Power of Your Subconscious Mind*. Englewood Cliffs, N.J., Prentice-Hall, Inc., 1963.

Peale, Norman Vincent. *The Power of Positive Thinking*. Prentice-Hall, Inc. 1952.

Prather, Hugh. *I Touch the Earth, the Earth Touches Me*. New York. Doubleday, 1972.

Other books I drew from:

Bosnak, Robert. *A Little Course in Dreams*. Boston & London. Shambhala, 1986.

Branden, Nathaniel. *The Psychology of Self-Esteem*. New York: Bantam Books, Inc., 1969.

Carson, Richard. *Taming Your Gremlin*. New York: Harper & Row Publishers, Inc., 1986.

Dyer, Wayne W. *The Sky's the Limit*. New York: Simon & Schuster, 1980.

———*You'll See It When You Believe It*. New York: Avon Books, Inc., 1990.

———*Gifts From Eykis*. New York: Simon & Schuster, 1983.

Gendlin, Eugene T. *Focusing*. New York: Bantam Doubleday, 1981.

————*Let Your Body Interpret Your Dreams.* Wilmette, Il., Chiron Publications, 1987.

Hoff, Benjamin. *The Tao of Pooh.* New York: Penguin Books, 1982.

Jung, C. G. *Memories, Dreams, Reflections.* New York: Random House, 1965.

Kornfield, Jack and Breiter, Paul. *A Still Forest Pond.* Wheaton, Il., Quest Books, 1985.

Mellon, Nancy. *Storytelling & The Art of Imagination.* Rockport, MA., Element, Inc., 1992 (Republished as *The Art of Storytelling* 1998).

Peck, M. Scott. *The Road Less Traveled.* New York: Simon and Schuster, 1978.